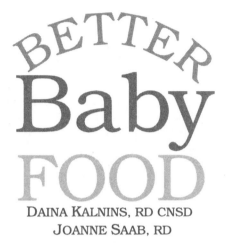

BETTER Baby FOOD

DAINA KALNINS, RD CNSD
JOANNE SAAB, RD

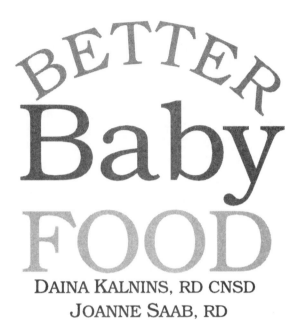

BETTER Baby FOOD

DAINA KALNINS, RD CNSD
JOANNE SAAB, RD

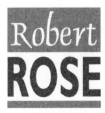

Robert
ROSE

Better Baby Food

For complete cataloguing information, see page 6.

DESIGN, EDITORIAL AND PRODUCTION:	MATTHEWS COMMUNICATIONS DESIGN INC.
COVER ILLUSTRATION:	SHARON MATTHEWS
MANAGING EDITOR:	PETER MATTHEWS
INDEXER:	BARBARA SCHON
COVER SCAN:	POINTONE GRAPHICS

We acknowledge the financial support of the Government of Canada through the Book Publishing Industry Development Program (BPIDP) for our publishing activities.

Published by: Robert Rose Inc. • 120 Eglinton Ave. E, Suite 1000, Toronto, Ontario, Canada M4P 1E2   Tel: (416) 322-6552

Printed in Canada

3 4 5 6 7 CPL 06 05 04

Contents

A B C D E F G H I J K L M N O P Q R S T U V W X Y Z

National Library of Canada Cataloguing in Publication Data

IN THE U.S.A.

Kalnins, Daina
   Better baby food

For use in the United States.
Includes bibliographical references and index.
ISBN 0-7788-0027-X

1. Cookery (Baby foods).   2. Infants – Nutrition.   I. Saab, Joanne.   II. Hospital
for Sick Children.   III. Title.

TX740.K34 2001a   641.5'622   C2001-930016-6

IN CANADA

Kalnins, Daina
   Better baby food

For use in Canada.
Includes bibliographical references and index.
ISBN 0-7788-0030-X

1. Cookery (Baby foods).   2. Infants – Nutrition.   I. Saab, Joanne.   II. Hospital for
Sick Children.   III. Title.

TX740.K34 2001   641.5'622   C00-933343-6

Introduction

EVERY PARENT WANTS THEIR BABY TO GET THE BEST POSSIBLE NUTRITION – AND TO SHARE that unforgettable expression of wonder, delight or uncertainty when a baby explores new foods and taste sensations. After all, good food and nutrition are essential to a baby's healthy growth and development, and to creating the foundation for sound eating habits in later life. But most parents aren't nutritionists. And the important task of choosing and preparing the best possible foods can be a little overwhelming.

In this book, we offer accurate, easy-to-follow, information and guidance as well as delicious child-tested and approved recipes to help you provide a balanced diet for your family. The book can be used as a quick reference or as a source of more comprehensive nutritional information. We are sure it will help to make nutrition for you and your child a pleasant experience.

Our backgrounds in nutrition working at The Hospital for Sick Children have given us together over 20 years experience in pediatric nutrition and research. We are both Registered Dietitians, a designation that requires a university degree in science, as well as internship experience. In our professional lives, we have provided nutritional guidance for infants and children – both sick and healthy – as well as answered countless questions about food and nutrition from parents, co-workers, pediatricians and general practitioners. This book is the product of that observation and experience, combined with careful research, and the collaborative effort of colleagues.

In addition to our professional backgrounds, one of us (Daina), with a 2-year-old and 6-month-old at home, brings to this book her personal experience as a parent of young children.

We have tried to make this book as comprehensive as possible, and to answer questions about topics that include breast feeding, introduction of solids, and appropriate time to try table foods. We will guide you on concerns about stool patterns, and growth issues. The large variety of recipes will help you feed your child a balanced, healthy diet that can be enjoyed by the whole family.

We encourage you to have fun with the amazing development of your child-feeding, growing, in a healthy way.

– DK and JS

Acknowledgments

First we would like to thank the Hospital for Sick Children and Robert Rose Inc. for giving us the opportunity to write this book. It has been an amazing experience both on professional and personal levels. Thanks especially to Bob Dees at Robert Rose. To the editorial and design team at Matthews Communications Design Inc., thank you for making our words and recipes come to life on paper. Thank you to Cyndy Deguisti for your guidance throughout this project.

Thank you to Margaret Howard, who worked with us and contributed nearly half the recipes for this book. Marg, it was such a pleasure working with you and we look forward to future collaborations.

A special thank you to Dr. Deborah O'Connor, Dr. Paul Pencharz and Debbie Stone, who took time out of their busy schedules to review the text portion of the book and provide insight and constructive comments to ensure our information was as accurate and up to date as possible with current research and opinion.

Also to all of our friends, family and co-workers, who kindly contributed their favorite kid-friendly recipes, including Karen Kurilla, Lucy Dardarian, Christine Dunlop, Joanne Haines, Denise Hawman, Joyce Hawman, Joann Herridge, Inta Huns, Ilze Kalnins, Joanne Munro, Joanne Nijhuis, and Constance Saab.

A heartfelt thank you to our families, who helped test our recipes by chopping, cooking, and even baking! You tasted our recipes when they turned out and even when they didn't. Most of all, thank you for always supporting us in whatever we do. Thanks especially to David, Blair, Natali, Matt, Denise, Barry and Joyce Hawman, and Joanne Munro.

We would also like to thank our co-workers in the department of clinical dietetics at The Hospital for Sick Children, who provided us with information, reviewed our work and provided support, including Joan Brennan, Joann Herridge and Donna Secker. Also to Aneta Plaga, who helped ease the burden of typing when the deadline was looming near.

Throughout this project, many friends provided much appreciated advice and encouragement. Thank you Debbie O'Connor, Patrice Banton, Ted and Cathy Watson, Dr. Stan Zlotkin, Monica O'Reilly, Gord Munro, and Abbe Klores.

A huge thank you to Jaclyn Quigley who volunteered hours of her time inputting recipes, completing journal searches and helping out with the nutritional analyses. Thanks, Jackie, for all your help. You did a great job.

Also, thank you to Linda Chow who completed the nutritional analysis for over 200 recipes in this book. Thank you for being so patient as we tested and changed recipes. Your help was invaluable.

Joanne would also like to thank Daina for making this book such a memorable project to work together on. Your support, and friendship, as well as your experience and expertise, are greatly valued. I think we make a great team, and look forward to working together again soon.

From Daina, a sincere thank you to Joanne Saab, a good friend, colleague and co-author. Throughout the long phone conversations, emails and meetings, you have demonstrated over and over again your knowledge, professionalism and commitment to this book. I have really enjoyed our partnership, and like you, look forward to future collaborations. Thanks also for your patience and understanding when Matt or Natali, or both, weren't quite so willing to let go of their mom's attention.

Nutritional Advice in Brief

Here, in no particular order, we offer our top 8 recommendations for parents of infants and toddlers. Each provides references for additional information within the book.

1. Breast feeding is recommended for infants (see pages 11 to 20). Formula feeding is an adequate nutritional alternative (see pages 21 to 30), but does not provide the many immunological benefits of breast feeding.

2. Be sure to supervise children when new solid foods are introduced into their diet (see pages 42 to 44). Learn what measures to take in case of choking (see pages 43, 61 to 62).

3. Parents need to be educated on principles of good nutrition if they want to provide the most nutritious food choices for their children. They should understand the basic elements of food – such as protein, fat , carbohydrates, vitamins and minerals – and the role played by each (see pages 73 to 78).

4. Children should understand from an early age the importance of good nutrition and its effects on their growth and well-being (see pages 50, 54, 81). This will help to promote good eating habits later in life.

5. Commercially prepared foods can provide adequate nutrition, but homemade foods (see pages 36 to 37) should provide at least a portion of a child's diet – and that of the family as a whole. (This is why we felt it was important to include a wide variety of nutritious, tasty recipes in this book).

6. Ensure that your child's diet contains an adequate supply of iron-rich foods. Inadequate iron intake can affect their behavior, learning ability and general well-being (see page 42). Young children are particularly at risk of iron deficiency (see pages 75 to 77).

7. As much as possible, ensure that your child has ready access to a supply of cut-up fresh fruit and vegetables (see pages 43, 52). When these foods are at hand, they are more likely to be eaten as snacks. As well, increased fruit and vegetable consumption helps to boost fiber intake, which helps with digestion and reduces constipation.

8. Encourage your child by example to eat nutritious foods and to be physically active. Childhood obesity is on the rise. It is up to parents to help prevent this disease (see pages 80 to 81).

CHAPTER 1

Breast Milk

MOTHERS FACE MANY CHALLENGES IN CARING FOR A newborn. But preparing healthy, nutritionally balanced meals need not be one of them.

With breast milk, nature has provided the perfect food for your baby. It is very easy to digest and is designed to meet just about all of a healthy infant's nutritional requirements for the first 4 to 6 months of life. The only real exception is vitamin D, which may need to be given as a supplement, particularly in sun-deprived northern locations (see box, page 13). Also, infants who are born extremely premature, weighing less than 2 kg (4 lbs), must receive breast milk that is fortified with extra calories and nutrients.

Can breast milk help reduce the risk of allergies?

Recent research has shown that for infants with a high risk of allergies (for example, when one or both parents, or a sibling, have an allergy), prolonging breast feeding for a minimum of 4 to 6 months can decrease the child's risk of developing allergy. However, for those infants with no strong family history of allergy, there is no clear evidence that breastfeeding provides a similar protective effect.

As well as being an unequalled source of nutrition – and a wonderful way for mother and child to bond – breastfeeding offers a number of other significant benefits.

Enhanced immunity. Breast milk provides immunities that help infants to fight infection. Studies have shown that exclusively breastfed babies have lower rates of ear infections, lower respiratory tract infections and diarrhea (gastroenteritis).

Convenience and economy. Breastfeeding is very convenient, since it is possible to breastfeed anytime, anywhere. It is always fresh and costs nothing.

Cleanliness. Breast milk does not require preparation or sterilization techniques that are dependent on a clean water supply.

Better for mothers too. Breastfeeding stimulates production of the hormone oxytocin, which causes the uterus to contract (what medical types call "uterine involution") and helps it to return more quickly to its pre-pregnancy size. Research also suggests that breastfeeding may reduce the risk of breast cancer in later life.

When you shouldn't breast-feed

While breast milk is generally the best food for newborns, there are some cases where breastfeeding is not recommended. One example, although extremely rare (less than 1 in 60,000 births), is in cases of galactosemia, a condition in which infants are born unable to metabolize breast milk. More common examples are when the breast milk may pose a danger to the baby because the mother's health or lifestyle – for example, if she is HIV positive, has untreated active tuberculosis, or is using illegal drugs.

BETTER BABY FOOD

T I P

Many prescription and over-the-counter drugs are compatible with breast feeding. In most cases, the baby receives less than 1% of the maternal dose through breast milk. To find out which medications are safe, talk to your doctor or call The Hospital for Sick Children's "Motherrisk" hotline at 416-813-6780 or, toll-free, at 1-877-327-4636. *www. motherrisk.org*

The basics of breast milk

Breast milk develops in stages, with each providing an important component of the baby's nutrition.

Colostrum. This is the first milk produced by moms in the first few days of a newborn infant's life. Colostrum is colorless, often thick and sticky, and contains high amounts of anti-infective properties called *immunoglobulins*. It also helps babies pass their first stool, which is called *meconium*. Often only very small amounts of colostrum are produced in those first few days of life, which can be frustrating for mothers who expect a greater volume of milk. However, it is important for new moms to continue to breastfeed. The volume will typically increase by Day 3 or 4, as this first stage gives way to the production of mature milk.

BETTER BABY FOOD

T I P

When a mother's milk comes in, breasts may become so firm that the baby has difficulty latching on to the nipple. To make this easier, and to soften the areola (the area around the nipple), manually express some milk into the baby's mouth.

Mature milk. This milk consists of two different components: *foremilk*, which is the milk a baby receives at the beginning of any feeding; and *hindmilk*, which is produced during each feed as the pressure in a mother's breasts decreases.

• Foremilk has a high water and sugar content, and quenches a baby's thirst. It is produced between feeds in response to previous suckling.

• Hindmilk, by contrast, is rich in fat and calories, and is produced during each feed as the pressure in the breast decreases. To ensure the infant receives this calorically dense milk, mothers should breastfeed until the baby pulls away or begins to nibble at the breast or when the infant falls asleep at the breast and doesn't start to feed again if milk is squeezed into its mouth. (See "How much is enough", page 16, for more information on feeding techniques.) Signs that a baby is

Topping up the vitamin D

A mother can have a well-balanced diet, and produce all the vitamins and minerals required to nourish an exclusively breastfed infant for up to six months. But even then, her breast milk may not contain enough vitamin D to prevent deficiency.

Vitamin D is a fat-soluble vitamin produced by the body in the presence of adequate sunlight. It is important for the development of healthy bones and teeth. Inadequate vitamin D intake can result in rickets, a condition in which bones become soft and can eventually bend.

Both the American and Canadian Pediatric Societies recommend that breastfed babies receive a daily vitamin D supplement of 400 IU (international units) for their first 6 months, until an adequate dietary source of vitamin D is introduced through other foods (such as cow's milk). Breastfed babies living in northern Canadian communities (or in Alaska) should receive 800 IU per day. Parents can purchase a vitamin D supplement appropriate for newborn infants (typically a liquid, dispensed with a 1 mL dropper) at any local pharmacy.

not receiving sufficient hind milk include frequent feeding, inadequate weight gain, and explosive production of green stools instead of the yellow, seedy-textured type. (See chart, page 17.)

Breast milk to go

In an ideal world, mothers would always be available to breastfeed their babies. But the realities of life often make this impossible. For such occasions, it is important to have a supply milk that has been expressed from the breast and is available for whenever the baby is hungry.

CHOOSING A BREAST PUMP. While it's possible to express breast milk manually, the task is considerably easier with a breast pump. There are many different types of breast pumps available, ranging from simple hand-operated models (costing between $20 and $80, depending on quality) to electric or battery-powered pumps designed for home use (between $90 and $120). The most powerful and efficient of all are professional- or hospital-grade electric pumps, which are prohibitively expensive to purchase but can be rented from some hospitals, pharmacies or medical supply companies at a nominal cost. Your birth hospital should be able to provide details. You can also contact Hollister Ltd. (a breastfeeding equipment manufacturer) or Medela Inc. to locate a supplier of breast pumps available for rental in your community. (For contact information, see "Resources" on page 20.) Finally, for Internet-enabled moms, it is now possible to shop for breast pumps on-line. Before you buy, however, compare the cost of purchasing a home-use pump against that of renting a professional-grade device. Depending on how often you expect to use a pump, one option may be significantly less expensive than the other.

BETTER BABY FOOD

T I P

Infants who are born extremely premature can be breastfed, although the breast milk will generally need to be fortified with extra calories and nutrients.

PREPARING AND USING A BREAST PUMP. Before pumping breast milk, be sure to wash your hands thoroughly with soap and water. Breast milk is relatively free of bacteria, but care must be taken not to contaminate the breast milk with bacteria from hands or dirty equipment. Breast pump kits should also be washed well with hot soapy water and air dried. Follow the manufacturer's instructions for sterilizing the pump, which is usually done on a daily basis. Mothers should pump each breast for 10 to 15 minutes or until milk stops flowing. Pumping should be done as often as a mother would breast-feed her infant – every 2 or 3 hours for newborns, with longer periods between feedings for older infants.

STORING EXPRESSED MILK. After using the breast pump, expressed milk should be stored in the refrigerator or freezer in sterile glass or hard plastic containers. Another option is to use plastic freezer bags that have been specially designed for freezing breast milk. (You can also use ordinary freezer bags, although these should be double-bagged to avoid punctures.) Once milk is collected in sterile containers, it should be labeled clearly with the date and time of expression so that the milk can be consumed by the baby in the order it was pumped. Frozen breast milk should be stored in small (2- to 4-oz) portions, since these will defrost quickly and less will be wasted if baby doesn't drink the entire amount of thawed milk. When freezing breast milk, be sure to leave some space at the top of the storage container as the milk will expand during freezing. Fresh breast milk can be stored for up to 48 hours in the refrigerator, and up to 6 months in the freezer if frozen using the proper techniques.

BETTER BABY FOOD

T I P

Once thawed, frozen breast milk should be refrigerated and consumed within 24 hours. Do not freeze again.

DEFROSTING FROZEN BREAST MILK. Defrosting should be done overnight in a refrigerator, where it will take approximately 8 to 12 hours to thaw completely. For parents in a hurry, frozen milk can be placed under warm running water or in a dish of warm water. Do not use boiling water, since this can destroy the milk's immunological (infection-fighting) properties. Breast milk should never be heated in a microwave, which changes the composition of breast milk and can cause "hot spots" that could burn the baby's mouth.

BREAST MILK EXPRESS
8 steps to success

1. Wash hands and equipment thoroughly.

2. If you are at work or away from your baby, find a quiet place to pump. An article of clothing or a blanket that smells like baby may help let down the milk.

3. Pump – approximately 10 to 15 minutes per breast until empty.

4. Collect milk in sterilized containers. Label clearly with date and time.

5. Freeze or refrigerate for later use.

6. Defrost frozen milk overnight in refrigerator or run under warm running water. Do not microwave or place breast milk in hot water. Test temperature before using.

7. Feed baby.

8. Discard any breast milk that remains after feeding.

BETTER BABY FOOD
T I P

If you alternate breasts between feedings, it's often helpful to attach a safety pin to the corresponding bra strap to remind you which breast was used.

How often and how long should you breastfeed?

Newborn infants should feed on cue about 8 to 12 times per day until satisfied. They will usually breastfeed for 10 to 15 minutes per breast at each feeding, although this time typically decreases as the baby gets older and learns to feed more efficiently. If a newborn infant, in the first few weeks of life, is not demanding to be fed at least every 4 hours, they should be awakened to feed. Crying is a late sign that an infant is hungry. Other signs or "cues" that an infant is ready to feed include increased fussiness or agitation, tongue or lip movements, fists in mouth, or opening their mouths when the skin around their mouth, cheeks or lips is touched.

How much is enough?

Newborns. The best way to know if a newborn infant is receiving enough breast milk is by counting the number of wet (or otherwise filled) diapers produced in a day. Weight gain is another. A newborn infant should have 6 to 8 wet diapers a day after the first week of life. During the first days of life wet diapers may be fewer. For example, on Days 1 to 3 of life infants may only have 3 wet diapers in a day. Wet dia-pers should increase in frequency and volume each day.

On Day 4 and 5, there should be 4 to 5 wet diapers. These diapers should be quite heavy and wet. Babies should also have about 3 to 5 stools per day. Babies should breast feed on cue (or demand), about 8 to 12 times per day (that is, every 1 1/2 to 2 hours). There may be a longer period during the night if the baby feeds frequently during the day.

Length of time spent at the breast is also a good indicator that your baby is receiving enough breast milk. Babies spend about 10 to 15 minutes per breast and should not routinely be falling asleep at the breast without feeding. While the baby feeds, there should be a rhythmic suckling and you should hear the baby swallowing. After feeding, breasts should feel softer.

To ensure adequate weight gain, be sure to have your baby prop-erly weighed (not on a home scale) after the first week (Day 7).

Eating and sleeping

Most parents are grateful for newborn infants who like to sleep. But sleepy babies are often hard to feed for more than 5 or 10 minutes before they nod off. To encourage longer feeding and ade-quate nutrition, newborns can be kept awake by tick-ling their toes or undressing them slightly.

WHEN TO GET HELP
4 signs that you need assistance with breastfeeding your baby

1. Baby has fewer than 2 soft stools per day in the first month.

2. Baby has dark urine and produces fewer than 3 wet diapers on Days 1 to 3, and fewer than 6 wet diapers by Day 5 or 6.

3. Baby is unusually sleepy and difficult to wake for feedings.

4. Baby is feeding less often than 8 times per 24 hours.

Older infants. Between the ages of 1 to 4 months, babies will feed less frequently than newborns – in most cases, between 6 to 8 times a day (or every 3 to 4 hours). They may also begin to sleep through the night (or longer) without feeding. Throughout this period, the infant should continue to produce 6 or more heavy, soaked diapers per day. Stool frequency varies between babies, but may be 3 to 5 daily. Weight gain provides a good indicator that the older infant is getting enough nutrition from breast feeding. Ask to see your baby's growth chart at his or her next doctor's appointment.

WHAT GOES IN, WHAT COMES OUT
Determining whether your NEWBORN is getting enough breast milk

DAYS AFTER BIRTH	NUMBER OF FEEDS	STOOLS	WET DIAPERS
1 to 2	Number of feeds will increase each day. Should feed 8 to 12 times/day	Dark green or black meconium. May only have 1 sticky stool	1 to 3 wet diapers, increasing in fullness each day*
3 to 4	8 to 12 times per day, every 2 to 3 hours	Day 3 stool may still be black. Day 4 stool will be lighter (yellowish) in color	3 or 4 soaked diapers *Note: Occasional brick-red staining is normal in Days 1 to 3.*
5 to 6	8 to 12 times per day	Minimum of 2 to 3 bowel movements per day. Stools will be odorless, a few tablespoons in volume and yellow/seedy in color and texture	6 or more, heavy soaked diapers. Will continue to have this many diapers for many months

When to wean your infant

There are many factors to consider when deciding when to wean an infant off the breast, including a mother's decision to return to the workforce (although many mothers are able to continue breastfeeding at work) and/or the baby's preference for finger foods or sip cups after these have been introduced to the diet. It is normal for mothers to continue breastfeeding until the infant is transitioned to whole milk at 9 to 12 months or even longer. If an infant is weaned off the breast prior to the introduction of whole milk, both the American and Canadian Pediatric Societies, recommends the use of an iron-fortified, cow's-milk-based infant formula as your best alternative to breastfeeding. (See Chapter 2, pages 21 to 22.)

Breastfeeding Q&A

Q. *Will skipping a breastfeed or prolonging the time between pumping increase my milk supply?*

A. Many mothers believe that skipping a feeding or prolonging the time between pumping will build their milk supply. In fact, the opposite is true. Skipping feeds sends a message to the mother's body that it has produced enough milk and does not need to produce more.

Q. *My pumped breast milk is often a different color on different days. Is there something wrong?*

A. The color, consistency and odor of breast milk can vary depending on many things, including the foods you eat. If you are freezing your breast milk, different foods found in your refrigerator or freezer can also affect the odor of your breastmilk.

Q. *Is it all right to give my breastfed baby a bottle? I've heard that it can lead to something called "nipple confusion."*

A. The mechanisms of breastfeeding and bottle feeding are quite different. If a baby is offered a bottle too soon – that is, before breastfeeding is well established – it is possible for a baby to develop "nipple confusion." This happens when a baby is unable to learn both techniques of breast and bottle feeding. This can result in inefficient sucking at the breast. By delaying the introduction of a bottle until breastfeeding is well established (about 4 weeks), nipple confusion can be avoided.

Q. *I am breastfeeding and taking many vitamin and herbal supplements. Could this be harmful to my baby?*

A. While there are many medications and supplements that can be taken while breastfeeding, there are some that should not be used. Herbal supplements, for example, should be avoided or used with caution while breastfeeding. Vitamins can also pass through to breast milk. So while a single multivitamin taken every day is beneficial to many mothers, this may not be the case if a number of vitamins are taken at once. This is especially true for single-vitamin preparations. For example, excess vitamin D supplementation has been reported to cause vitamin D toxicity in breastfed infants. Your doctor, pharmacist or dietitian can guide you about specific supplements.

For more infant-related Q & As, see Chapter 2, page 29.

Resources

- La Leche League International   www.lalecheleague.org

- Medela Inc. 815-363-1166 (USA) or 1-800-435-8316 (Canada)   www.medela.com

- Hollister Ltd. 1-800-323-4060 (USA) or 1-800-263-7400 (Canada)   www.hollister.com

- www.breastfeeding.com

- Motherrisk 416-813-6780 or 1-877-327-4636 (toll free)   www.motherrisk.org

- Your local birth hospital or public health unit

CHAPTER **2**

Infant Formula

WHILE BREAST MILK IS GENERALLY ACCEPTED TO BE the best food for newborns (as discussed in Chapter 1), there may be some circumstances in which a mother will, having considered the alternatives, choose not to breast feed. Here the most acceptable alternative is to give the baby a cow's-milk-based infant formula until he or she is 9 to 12 months old and begins to drink conventional whole milk.

With so many different types of formula available in the marketplace today, new parents may find it difficult to know which is the most appropriate choice for their child. The good news is that the composition of infant formula is subject to strict regulations, so you can be confident that just about any choice will provide nutrition that is, if not quite equal to that of breast milk, at least similarly balanced.

Is that formula fortified?

While most formulas will state quite clearly on their packaging whether or not they are iron fortified, some may not. If you are unsure, read the nutritional analysis on the label. Iron-fortified formulas must contain 1 mg iron per 100 kcal (about 6.8 mg per 1 L). Non-fortified formulas are still required to contain at least 0.15 mg iron per 100 kcal.

Formula fundamentals

While all types of infant formula are intended to provide good nutrition, they differ according to the food source on which they are based. These are described below.

Cow's-milk-based formula. (*examples: Enfalac, Enfamil with Iron, Similac Advance*). This is the most common type of infant formula on the market – and the best choice for healthy term (that is, not premature) infants who have no family history of allergy. These formulas come in both low-iron and iron-fortified varieties. The low-iron type is designed to mimic the iron content of breast milk. However, for non-breastfed infants who will be consuming formula exclusively until they are 9 to 12 months old (when they have transitioned to whole milk and other foods), most health authorities recommend using iron-fortified formula. This is based on the fact that between the ages of 4 and 6 months, formula-fed infants will have depleted their own body's iron stores and will require additional iron from the foods they eat. Although low-iron formulas do contain small amounts of iron, the quantity may be insufficient to prevent deficiency in infants over 6 months of age.

Soy-based formulas *(examples: Prosobee, Isomil, Alsoy).* Parents choose soy-based formulas for a number of reasons – many having to do with their own dietary preferences. For example, they may be strict vegetarians (vegans). They may have an allergy (real or perceived) to dairy. And they may interpret symptoms such as loose stools, vomiting and colic as evidence of a similar allergy in their newborn. In fact, there are comparatively few cases where the use of a soy-based formula is medically necessary. These include cases of *galactosemia*, a disorder in which infants are unable to digest the carbohydrate galactose.

Still, it has become common practice to prescribe soy formula for children with cow's milk protein allergy. This practice is generally not recommended. Why? Because there is a significant body of research data to suggest that, of infants with cow's milk allergy, some will also have an allergy to soy protein. Where cow's milk allergy is a real concern, an alternative may be a hypoallergenic formula (such as Nutramigen), in which the protein is extensively broken down. (See following page for details.)

Although soy formulas are not recommended as the first choice for healthy term infants who are not being breast fed, the American Academy of Pediatrics suggests that soy protein-based formulas are safe and effective alternatives to breast milk or cow's milk based formulas to provide appropriate nutrition for normal growth and development.

Does soy affect hormonal development?

In recent years, soy formulas have become the subject of considerable media attention because they contain phyto-estrogens – naturally occurring compounds that have estrogen-like activity. It has been suggested that these compounds may affect the development of an infant's hormonal (or endocrine) system. And, in fact, a recent study showed that infants consuming soy formulas did have higher levels of phyto-estrogens in their blood. The significance of this finding remains unclear. In Canada, for example, soy formulas have been routinely used for 40 years with no evidence of adverse hormone-related effects.

BETTER BABY FOOD

T I P

Lactose-free formulas are not appropriate for infants with galac-tosemia, a disorder in which infants cannot digest the sugar galac-tose, since they contain residual galactose.

Protein hydrolysate formulas, casein-based (example: *Nutramigen*). This type of formula is considered to be hypoallergenic, which, as noted earlier, is a better choice for non-breastfed infants who have a confirmed allergy to cow's milk protein. (Of course, as we have also mentioned previously, breast milk poses the least risk for children at high risk of developing allergy.) Here the protein is broken down into very small units called *peptides* and *free amino acids*. Although less palatable to some infants, this type of formula is generally well-accepted by those whose sense of taste is not well developed. This type of formula is also very expensive.

Protein hydrolysate formulas, whey-based (example: *Good Start*). This type of formula contains proteins that have been slightly broken down to form smaller incomplete proteins. The proteins are still quite large, however, so this formula is not appropriate for children with a confirmed allergy to cow's milk protein. It is uncertain whether the formula is suitable for those children at high risk of milk allergy (that is, where a parent or sibling is allergic). The formula offers the benefits of being similar in taste and having a cost comparable to that of standard cow's-milk-based formula.

Lactose-free formulas (example: *Enfalac Lactose Free*). Lactose-free formulas are based on cow's milk, but have had the lactose removed and replaced with corn syrup solids. They are intended for infants who are unable to digest lactose, a carbohydrate (sugar) found in cow's milk. These infants, described as having primary lactose intolerance, are actually quite rare. More common are children who develop a temporary version of this condition, called secondary lactose intolerance, which typically accompanies an episode of diarrhea. Lactose-free formulas can also be useful in these cases, providing nutrition until the diarrhea subsides and the ability to digest lactose returns.

Follow-up formulas *(examples: Nestle Follow Up, Nestle Follow-Up Soy, Enfalac/Enfamil Next Step)*. These formulas are intended for older infants between the ages of 6 to 12 months. They are a better choice than whole cow's milk for children at an age where they can benefit from different proportions of nutrients, including calories, iron and essential fatty acids. These formulas also have a lower renal solute load than whole cow's milk (see page 26 for details), and are therefore easier on a baby's kidneys. This type of product can be based on cow's milk or soy; both varieties are iron-fortified. While follow-up formulas claim to offer benefits over traditional infant formulas, this has not been proved. Parents can comfortably use the same "starter" formula from birth until 12 months of age.

Added-rice formulas *(example: Enfalac AR)*. For otherwise healthy infants who occasionally spit up, this product combines rice starch and a conventional cow's-milk-based formula. The starch is intended to help the formula remain settled in the child's stomach. If your child spits up persistently, you should see your family physician or pediatrician for further recommendations.

Specialty formulas *(examples: Pregestimil, Alimentum, Portagen, and Neocate)*. Specialty formulas are available for those infants who have problems with digestion and/or absorption of carbohydrates, protein, fat, or other nutrients. These formulas are generally used in a hospital setting under the supervision of a dietitian and doctor. They are the most expensive formulas available. If your child is on a specialty formula, and you have questions, contact your dietitian or pediatrician for more information.

Powder, liquid, or ready to use?

Formulas are typically sold as concentrates (powdered or liquid) that must be mixed with water before using, or in premixed form. While their nutritional content remains the same for any given type of formula, they are significantly different in terms of cost and convenience

Powdered concentrate is the least expensive type of formula (see chart, below). It must be measured and mixed with clean water. (Use sterilized water for children under 4 months.) Once opened, a tin can be stored for up to 1 month before discarding.

FORM AND SUBSTANCE
Determining which form of infant formula is best for you

FORM	PROS	CONS
Powdered concentrate	Cost (see next page) Keeps for 1 month after opening	Risk of measuring error
Liquid concentrate	Easy to measure Easy to mix	Must be used within 48 hours of opening
Ready-to-use	No mixing Convenient Not reliant on water supply	Cost (see next page)

Liquid concentrate is easier to measure and mix than the powdered variety, and is typically 30 to 40% more expensive. It's shelf-life is also considerably shorter: once opened, a container of unmixed formula must be used within 48 hours. (Formula that has been mixed with water must be used up or thrown out within 24 hours.)

Ready-to-use formula offers the greatest convenience, since it requires no mixing and does not depend on having a clean water supply (which can be useful when traveling). Convenience has a cost, however, since this is by far the most expensive way to buy formula – up to 4 times as costly as powdered concentrate. While all types of formula are available in powdered form (and most types as liquid), ready-to-use formats are typically offered only for cow's-milk- and soy-based formulas.

So which format to choose? Ultimately, that will depend on your budget, time constraints and personal preference.

COUNTING THE COST
How different types of formula compare

FORMULA TYPE	Relative Cost		
	POWDER	LIQUID	READY-TO-USE
Cow's-milk-based	Low	Moderate	Very High
Lactose-free CMB	Moderate	Moderate	N/A
Soy-based	Moderate	Moderate to High	Very High
Follow-up	Moderate	Moderate	N/A
Protein hydrolysate (Nutramigen)	Very High	N/A	N/A

Milk by any other name

So how does formula compare with breast milk? How does it compare with whole cow's milk? As noted earlier and as shown in the chart on page 27, formula manufacturers attempt to provide the same nutritional balance as breast milk. Comparing breast milk with cow's-milk-based formula, we see that the distribution of calories from carbohydrates and fat are roughly the same, although proteins are slightly higher in formula.

In the case of whole cow's milk, however, we see a dramatically higher protein content than is found in either formula or breast milk. This is why whole milk is not recommended for infants before the age of 9 months. The excess protein (and salt) in cow's milk creates what is called a high *renal solute load*, which means that these nutrients can be difficult for an infant's kidneys to process.

By avoiding cow's milk during the first 9 months, infants give their kidneys a chance to develop to the point where they are able to handle this additional protein. If consumed at a younger age – say, before 6 months – cow's milk can cause a variety of problems, which can include bleeding in the digestive tract.

Cow's milk is also very low in iron, which is another reason to avoid giving it to infants before the age of 9 months. If is introduced earlier – that is, before the infant is consuming a variety of foods (including iron-fortified rice cereal and meat) – he or she could be at risk of developing *iron-deficiency anemia*. (This condition is discussed in greater detail in Chapter 7; see pages 75 to 76.)

LIQUID ASSETS
Comparing the nutrient composition of milk and formula

	BREAST MILK	COW'S MILK-BASED FORMULA	WHOLE COW'S MILK
Protein	6%	8 to 9%	20%
Fat	50%	45 to 50%	50%
Carbohydrates	40 to 45%	41 to 43%	30%

Preparing and using formula

Sterilize. Before preparing formula, it is important to sterilize all bottles, nipples and caps (particularly important for infants younger than 4 months old). To do this, all equipment should be boiled for 5 minutes.

Boil the water. Most domestic water supplies contain at least some bacteria that may be harmful to an infant – again, particularly when the baby's age is less than 4 months. To ensure that the water is sterile it should be boiled for 2 minutes, then allowed to cool until lukewarm, before preparing the formula according to the package instructions.

Use it or lose it. Once prepared, formula can be stored in the refrigerator for up to 24 hours, after which any unused formula should be discarded.

For more information on infant feeding, see Chapter 1.

How much formula is enough?

Unlike breastfeeding, where it is difficult for mothers to know exactly how much a baby is drinking, it is possible to measure an infant's formula intake. The volume of formula consumed will increase with age and will vary depending on size and activity. The following chart gives an example of estimated intake:

AGE	FEEDS/DAY	QUANTITY/FEED*
Birth to 1 week	6 to 10	2 to 3 oz (60 to 90 mL)
1 week to 1 month	6 to 8	3 to 4 oz (90 to 120 mL)
1 to 3 months	5 to 6	4 to 6 oz (120 to 180 mL)
3 to 7 months	4 to 5	6 to 7 oz (180 to 210 mL)
7 to 12 months	3 to 4	7 to 8 oz (210 to 240 mL)

* Values are approximate; actual intake will vary with infant's size and activity level.

Formula **Q&A**

Q. *Which formula is best? There are so many to choose from.*

A. In cases where the mother decides not to breastfeed, virtually all pediatricians and dietitians recommend a cow's-milk-based, iron-fortified formula as the next best choice for healthy, full term babies with no family history of allergy. Nutritionally, it does not matter if it is powder, liquid concentrate or ready to use. These choices must be made based on affordability and lifestyle. See pages 25 to 26 for more information.

Q. *My 2-month-old daughter spits up a lot. I have heard that adding infant rice cereal to her formula may help. Is this true?*

A. Many pediatricians do suggest adding a small amount of rice cereal to a bottle of formula or expressed breast milk (1 to 2 tbsp [15 to 25 mL] per 1/2 cup [125 mL]) to help with spitting up. However, research has not proven that the addition of rice cereal will always be effective. If spitting up is a problem for your infant, seek further advice from your doctor or pediatrician.

Q. *My newborn son is now 7 days old and still has not regained his birth weight. Is this okay?*

A. Newborns may lose up to 10% of their birth weight in the first few days of life. By Day 10 to 14, however, infants should regain their birth weight. Not all infants will regain their birth weight in the same amount of time, but if by Day 14 your infant has not regained his or her birth weight you should talk to your doctor.

Q. *How do I know if my child is gaining weight as she should?*

A. The best way to know for sure if your child is gaining weight and growing normally is to ask you doctor to see her growth chart. This data is the product of extensive research on the growth of thousands of children over time and will determine whether your child's weight is appropriate in relation to her length. As a rule of thumb, infants should double their birth weight by 4 to 6 months and triple their birth weight by 1 year. Birth length should increase by about 50% after 1 year.

Resources

- Mead Johnson   www.meadjohnson.com

- Nestle   www.verybestbaby.com

- Wyeth   www.wyethnutritionals.com

- Ross   www.ross.com/html/unifiedsite.cfm

CHAPTER **3**

Introducing Solids
(4 to 8 months)

A DIET OF BREAST MILK (OR FORMULA) IS ALL A BABY NEEDS for the first 3 or 4 months. In fact, before then, an infant's digestive system is unprepared to handle anything else. After this period, however, it is important to start introducing the solid foods that will provide your baby with the nutrients he or she needs for proper growth and development.

When your grandparents started

Before the 1920s, babies seldom started solids until 12 months. But in 1930, with the development of Pablum (an infant rice cereal) at the Hospital for Sick Children, this practice began to change. Until the 1970s, the accepted wisdom was to introduce solids (primarily fruits and vegetables) at 6 months. Today, however, most health authorities recommend starting solids as early as 4 months, usually beginning with a single-ingredient, iron-fortified grain cereal.

When to begin

There is no magic time at which the introduction to solids must take place. Each child grows and develops at a different rate. So while one may be developmentally advanced enough to start solids at 4 months, another may not be ready until 5 months. Ultimately, the decision to start must be individualized.

While the time to start introducing solids will vary between children, 4 months is generally accepted as being suitable. By this age, the digestive tract is mature enough to digest complex proteins, fats and carbohydrates. In addition, 4 months is about the time when most infants are able to sit (if supported) and are physically able to swallow non-liquid foods. (Younger babies have what is called an extrusion reflex, which prevents them from swallowing – and possibly choking on – solids; this reflex disappears between 4 and 6 months.) A 4-month-old also has the motor skills necessary to accept non-liquid foods – such as the ability to close the lips over a spoon when it is removed from his or her mouth.

MEALTIME MILESTONES
When and what an infant is able to eat

AGE	DEVELOPMENT	FOODS
Birth to 4 months	Digestive system lacks enzymes to process solids	Breast milk
	Unable to swallow non- liquid foods	Infant formula
4 to 6 months	Able to sit if supported	Breast milk
	Can grasp objects (such as a bottle); able to close lips around a spoon	Iron-fortified Infant formula Infant cereal (diluted)
	Able to indicate hunger/ fullness	Strained fruits and vegetables
6 to 9 months	Able to sit unsupported	Breast milk
	Improved ability to grasp and manipulate objects	Infant formula
	Begins to develop ability to chew	Infant cereal
	Teething begins	Puréed meats Plain yogurt, grated cheese

It is important to remember that solids must be introduced gradually. During the 5- or 6-month transition period, breast milk or formula will continue to be your baby's primary source of nutrition. Also during this time, an infant's skills will continue to develop. At 4 to 6 months, babies typically learn to grasp a bottle (or spoon, for breastfed babies), as well as other objects. At 5 to 6 months, they are able to express hunger by opening their mouths and sitting forward when food is presented to them. Conversely, they are also able to show disinterest in food (or fullness) by leaning back in their highchair, pushing food away with hands, or turning their face away from what is being offered. Between 7 and 9 months, the ability to chew solid foods begins to develop.

Steps to
solid foods

Don't wait too long

While many parents recognize the importance of not starting solids too soon, they may not realize that it's also possible to start too late. Research has shown that if a child is not introduced to solids before 9 months, he or she may have difficulty accepting textures later.

BETTER BABY FOOD

T I P

New foods should be introduced one at a time with a couple of days in between each new food offered. This enables parents to identify which foods are not tolerated well by their infant.

BETTER BABY FOOD

T I P

When introducing solids, stool color and frequency may change. The amount produced will sometimes decrease and have a more pungent smell – particularly in the case of breastfed babies.

As noted earlier, the transition to solid foods is intended to satisfy hunger and to provide a nutritional complement to your baby's liquid diet. Over time, as more solids are introduced, the intake of breast milk or formula will decrease accordingly. Let's take a look at the types of solid foods in order of introduction.

Step 1: Cereals and Grains

It is generally recommended that a baby's first solid food be a single-ingredient, iron-fortified grain cereal. The single-ingredient composition is important, since this makes it easy to identify the source of any allergic reaction. And because such a reaction is least likely to occur with rice, your first choice should be a rice-based infant cereal.

Iron-fortification is no less important. Between 4 and 6 months, an infant's own iron stores will become depleted, after which the iron must be supplemented from the diet. This is particularly true for infants who are exclusively breast fed, or whose infant formula is not iron-fortified.

The infant cereal should be mixed to a thin applesauce-like texture and fed to the baby with an infant-sized spoon. An infant beginning solids for the first time will take approximately 2 to 3 teaspoons (10 to 15 mL) once daily, and progress in volume from there.

Once you are certain that your baby is able to digest a rice-based cereal, you can start introducing other single-ingredient cereals, including those based on barley or oats. Each new type of cereal should be tried over a number of days to ensure that it does not cause an allergic reaction. Finally, if no adverse reaction occurs (such as hives, rash, sudden vomiting or diarrhea; see page 63), you may wish to try a mixed cereal.

Bottles are for liquids only

Some parents believe that adding a little infant cereal to their baby's bottle is the best way to introduce the texture of solid foods. This is not recommended, since adding cereal to liquid actually dilutes the texture of the food and can interfere with the development of an infant's feeding skills.

Lima beans? Yuck!

Sure, you may have an aversion to certain types of vegetables. But your baby doesn't. So try to avoid letting your personal tastes interfere with what veggies and fruit you choose to serve. Believe it or not, your reaction (including words and/or facial expressions) can have a profound effect upon an infant's willingness to try and enjoy new foods.

Step 2: Vegetables and Fruit

Between the ages of 6 and 7 months, your baby should be ready to start eating strained vegetables and fruit. Not only do these foods add taste, texture, color and variety to an infant's expanding diet, they are also good sources of vitamins A and C. As with the grains, introduce a new food every few days, satisfying yourself that it is well tolerated, before moving on to the next.

Don't rush the veggies

Some types of strained vegetables and fruits — including spinach, beets, turnips, carrots, green beans, mixed vegetables and bananas – contain nitrates, and should therefore not be given to infants younger than 4 months. In sufficient concentrations, nitrate can cause these children to develop methemoglobinemia, a condition in which blood cells do not transport oxygen efficiently. After the age of 6 months, however, vegetables and fruits do not pose a risk, since infants are then able to handle nitrates in their diet.

Should you start your baby with fruits or vegetables? Some authorities believe that it is better to have an infant become accustomed to vegetables before introducing sweet-tasting fruits. But this is not always true. In fact, some infants who start exclusively with vegetables may refuse fruit later on. Like adults, infants have their own likes and dislikes. Try a variety of fruits and vegetables, perhaps alternating the introduction of one fruit with one vegetable. Nutritionally, it makes no difference, since breast milk or formula supplies most of the infant's nutrients at this stage.

Start with a few tablespoons of either a puréed vegetable or fruit, served twice a day. All vegetables and fruits are good choices, including strained sweet potato, peas, squash, pears, apples and bananas.

Step 3: Meat and Alternatives

At 7 to 9 months, babies can be introduced to meats and alternatives – including puréed meat, fish, poultry, cooked egg yolks (not whites; see sidebar), legumes and tofu. These foods provide additional flavor and variety, as well as a good source of supplemental protein and, in the case of strained meats, an excellent source of iron.

Start by choosing from commercially prepared products such as strained chicken with broth, lamb with broth, or beef with broth. If your child is able to tolerate these well, you can move on to "vegetables and meat" mixtures, which contain less meat and fewer calories. (Check the label to see which ingredient is listed first; that will be primarily what's in the jar.) Of course, as an alternative to buying prepared plain meats with broth, you can always make your own (see page 155).

Step 4: Milk and Milk Products

At around the same time that you introduce your child to meats and alternatives (7 to 9 months), you can also start adding milk products to his or her diet. Milk and milk products provide fat, protein and calcium. Start by giving your infant 1 to 2 tablespoons (15 to 25 mL) per day.

Good first-choices include plain yogurt, cottage cheese or grated hard cheeses. Although whole (homogenized) cow's milk can be introduced after 9 months, breast milk and iron-fortified formula are good choices for infants up to the age of 12 months. "Follow up" formulas, intended for infants over 6 months, are also preferable to cow's milk (from 6 to 9 months), although they do not offer any meaningful nutritional benefits over traditional "starter" formula.

Hold the egg whites

The introduction of egg whites should be delayed until an infant is at least 12 months old. Egg whites contain more than 20 different types of protein – all (or any one) of which can contribute to the development of an allergy or intolerance. (See pages 66 to 67 for more details.)

What about milk allergies?

Research shows that as many as 2 to 3% of infants have an allergy to cow's milk, although most grow out of it by the time they are 3 years old. Higher-risk babies – specifically, those whose parents and/or siblings have a milk allergy – should be checked by a physician before placing them on a milk-free diet. (See page 65 for more details.)

Foods	From **birth to 4** months	From **4 to 6** months	From **6 to 9** months	From **9 to 12** months
Breast Milk	Nursing on demand. Exclusively breastfed babies should receive a vitamin D supplement.	Nursing on demand. Exclusively breastfed babies should receive a vitamin D supplement.	Nursing on demand. Breastfed babies should receive a vitamin D supplement.	Nursing on demand.
Iron-fortified Formula	Formula feedings on demand, about 8 to 5 feedings every 24 hours. Boil all water for formula and drinking water.	Formula feedings on demand, about 6 to 4 feedings every 24 hours.	Formula feedings on demand, about 5 to 3 feedings every 24 hours.	Formula feedings or whole cow's milk, about 4 to 3 feedings every 24 hours.
Iron-fortified Infant Cereal Other Grain Products	None	May start to introduce iron-fortified infant cereal - rice or barley. Mix with breast milk or formula. Feed cereal from a spoon, not from the bottle. Start with 2 to 3 teaspoons, progress to 2 to 4 tablespoons twice daily.	Continue with iron-fortified infant cereal, 2 to 4 tablespoons twice daily. Introduce other Grain Products like dry toast or unsalted crackers.	Continue with iron-fortified infant cereal. Introduce other plain cereals, bread, rice and pasta, 8 to 10 tablespoons a day.
Vegetables	None	None	Offer pured cooked vegetables - yellow, green or orange. Progress to soft mashed cooked vegetables, 4 to 6 tablespoons a day.	Offer mashed or diced cooked vegetables, 6 to 10 tablespoons a day.
Fruit	None	None	Offer pured cooked fruits, very ripe mashed fruit (e.g. banana) 6 to 7 tablespoons a day. Around 7 to 9 months fruit juice may be offered from a cup.	Offer soft fresh fruits, peeled, seeded and diced or canned fruits packed in water or juice, diced, 7 to 10 tablespoons a day.
Meat & Alternatives	None	None	After vegetables and fruit, offer pured cooked meat, fish, chicken, tofu, mashed beans, egg yolk, 1 to 3 tablespoons a day.	Offer minced or diced cooked meat, fish, chicken, tofu, beans, egg yolk, 3 to 4 tablespoons a day.
Milk Products	None	None	Offer plain yoghurt (3.25% MF or higher), cottage cheese or grated hard cheese, 1 to 2 tablespoons a day.	Introduce whole (homo) cow's milk. Progress from a bottle to a cup. Continue with plain yoghurt (3.25% MF or higher), cottage cheese or other cheese, 2 to 4 tablespoons a day.
Texture Other Advice	Milk from breast or bottle.	Runny, thin cereal from a spoon.	Thickened cereal. Finely mashed soft solids. Avoid egg white, added sugar, salt.	Soft minced or diced table foods. Avoid egg white, added sugar, salt.

Offer new foods in small amounts, one food at a time every few days. Try not to be restricted by your own food likes and dislikes. When you are sure that the new foods are well accepted by your baby, you can the feed mixtures of foods. Your baby will let you know whether you are giving enough to eat or drink.

Store-bought or homemade?

Are homemade baby foods better than the store-bought variety? Certainly, commercially prepared foods are more convenient; homemade baby foods, although not terribly complicated, are nevertheless time-consuming to make. Nutritionally, studies have not found significant differences between commercially or home prepared baby foods. Children have been shown to grow and develop equally well on both.

Where the two types of foods can differ is in the additives used – specifically, sugar, salt and modified starch, all of which are often found in many commercially prepared foods. Check labels for ingredients.

Sugar is sometimes used in baby desserts as a sweetener.

Salt is another common additive, although often more so in homemade baby foods than in commercial varieties. Why? Simply because parents tend to season foods to suit their own tastebuds, often forgetting that infant palates have not been similarly conditioned to need the flavor of salt. So if you decide to make your own baby food, remember to ease up on the salt shaker: What may taste bland to you may not taste bland to your infant.

Modified starch, typically based on corn or tapioca, is often added to commercial baby foods. These compounds act as stabilizers to provide a desired consistency, texture and shelf life, primarily in desserts and junior foods. Research has demonstrated that modified starch is not harmful, and is fairly well digested by infants.

While research suggests that there is nothing unhealthy about commercially prepared baby food, many parents simply prefer to make their own. The good news here is that, while time-consuming, home-prepared infant foods are actually quite simple to make. They are also less expensive and give parents precise control over the ingredients used.

For a variety of flavorful and nutritious first-solids recipes – including baby fruit, vegetables and meats – see pages 108 to 111, and page 155. These recipes can be made ahead of time and frozen in ice-cube trays, which divide the food into portion sizes that are ideal for a young infant. The amount of sugar used, if any, is controlled and the variety of home prepared foods is limitless. For example, commercially prepared asparagus or mango may be difficult to find on your grocery store shelves but can be prepared in your own kitchen with ease. Virtually any fruit, vegetable or meat found in the grocery store can be used to prepare your own baby foods.

Baby organics

Concerned about chemical residues in produce? Then you may want to consider organic baby food. These products are made from organically grown fruits and vegetables, which are free of pesticides. They are also, as you might expect, more expensive than traditional store-bought baby foods. Organic baby foods can also be prepared in your own home using organically grown produce.

Here come the teeth

Teething can begin as early as 3 months or as late as 1 year, but usually begins at around 6 to 8 months and lasts for about 2 years. The first teeth cut are usually the incisor or front lower, then upper teeth.

The pain of teething – and the irritability that can accompany it – varies from one child to the next. In some cases, the discomfort can affect a child's appetite, but typically for no longer than a day or two. Some relief can be obtained by giving your baby pain-relief medication, cool teething rings or bagels or crusts of bread. Be wary of using teething gels, however. These products are essentially surface anesthetics that numb the contact area. While intended for the gums only, these gels are often applied inadvertently to the tongue, which may cause a child to choke or be insensitive to hot foods. Check with your GP or pediatrician before using these products. (For more information on teething and tooth care, see pages 46 to 47.)

First Solids
Q&A

Q. *When is my child old enough to start solids?*

A. Children are ready at different times to start solids. On average, however, the usual age is somewhere between 4 and 6 months. Starting solids too early or too late can be detrimental. See pages 31 to 33 for more details.

Q. *My 4-month-old daughter hates the taste of rice cereal. What can I do?*

A. Infant rice cereal is often the first food given to babies, since rice is very unlikely to cause an allergic reaction and it is a great source of dietary iron. If your child appears to dislike the taste of rice cereal, try changing the temperature at which you serve it, or change the consistency by adding more or less liquid. Also, for a change in flavor, try preparing the cereal with water or breast milk or formula.

Q. *Will giving my 7-week-old son cereal at bedtime help him sleep through the night?*

A. Research has not shown that early introduction of cereals at bedtime will help babies sleep through the night. Babies generally begin to sleep through the night (8 consecutive hours) sometime after the age of 2 to 3 months, regardless of whether or not they are fed cereals at bedtime.

Q. *My 7-month-old son doesn't seem to like any of the strained fruits and vegetables I am offering him. What should I do?*

A. The first reaction of some babies to an unfamiliar food is to spit it back out. It is important to persist, however; keep offering the food for a few days to see if he or she will eventually accept it. Once a food has been tried for a few days without success, move on to another food. Also, try not to let your personal tastes (or, more importantly, distastes) affect the manner in which you present the food. No matter how unappetizing you may find them personally, always offer new foods with enthusiasm. (See page 34 for more details.)

Q. *Why should new foods be offered at intervals of at least 3 days?*

A. Solids should be introduced one at a time with about 3 days between each new food so that if an allergy or intolerance is to occur, it will be easy to identify which food is the cause.

Q. *Do I need to switch to a "follow-up" formula when my child is 6 months old?*

A. For growing infants at 6 months, "follow-up" formulas are a better choice than cow's milk, since they provide a superior balance of calories, iron and essential fatty acids. Compared to conventional starter formulas, however, these products offer no significant nutritive advantage. Starter formulas can be used until an infant is 12 months old.

Q. *My husband and I both had food allergies as young children and I am worried about starting solids for my 6-month-old infant. What should I do?*

A. Introducing single foods, one at a time every 3 days or so, will help you to identify any allergy if it occurs. Extending breast feeding is also helpful for reducing allergy risk, since it may give a young infant's digestive tract time to mature and develop the ability to exclude allergic molecules from causing a reaction. You may wish to delay the introduction of common sources of food allergies (such as cow's milk, eggs, and nuts) until your child is a little older. Ask your doctor for more advice on how long to delay the introduction of specific foods. (See pages 63 to 67 for more information on food allergies.)

Q. *Should I make my own baby food, or are commercial foods okay?*

A. If you have the time and desire to make your own baby food, then by all means do so. It provides a great opportunity to try some different fruits, vegetables and meats. But if you don't have the time or inclination, don't worry — commercially prepared baby foods are perfectly acceptable and offer comparably good nutrition. Just be sure to read the labels on store-bought baby foods. Some older toddler desserts may include unnecessary sugar. Beginner foods should not contain salt, preservatives or color.

Q. *My 7-month-old son is teething. What can I give him to soothe the pain?*

A. Teething can be a difficult time for both infant and parents. Acceptable methods for managing pain include acetaminophen drops or a cooled plastic teething ring. Biscuit or bagel pieces are also good choices. (See page 38.)

Resources

- Beech Nut Foods www.beechnut.com
- Gerber Baby Foods www.gerber.com
- Heinz Baby Foods www.heinzbaby.com (Canadian site); call 1-800-USA-BABY in America

CHAPTER **4**

Time for Table Food
(8 to 12 months)

B Y THE AGE OF 8 MONTHS, MANY INFANTS ARE ABLE TO PROGRESS from simple puréed or strained foods to more solid or textured table foods – pieces of bread, perhaps, or some soft vegetables or fruit. For parents and infants alike, this is a time of ongoing discovery, occasional frustration, and eventual reward.

Take cover!

Making the transition to textures can be (okay, is almost always) a messy business. It is at this stage that infants learn to handle food themselves, with the result that much of it will end up someplace other than in their mouths. So invest in a good bib – one with a water-resistant backing and a soft, easy-to-clean front. If you prefer, you can use a harder plastic bib with a "trap" in front to catch food. Either way, the bib should dry quickly after cleaning, so it is ready to use for the next meal. Or have a few handy so that a clean one is always available.

Ready for textures?

There is no specific time to make the transition to more textured food since, as we have stated previously (and no doubt will again), each child is different. Very often a parent will know when the child is ready – either intuitively or from previous experience. Sometimes the emergence of teeth is taken as an indication of readiness, although this does not always matter. As a rule, however, if an infant is able to eat small slices of soft food without gagging or choking, and clearly enjoys these types of foods, then they are ready. But if you have doubts, seek the advice of your pediatrician.

Ultimately, the decision must be one with which you are comfortable. If you are not ready to offer textured foods, then wait until you are. An infant will sense your anxiety, and a few extra weeks of purées will not make any difference.

Iron-clad nutrition

Iron plays a very important role in a child's development, and studies have shown that iron deficiency can affect a child's learning ability early on in life. Low iron can also leave a child pale, irritable and tired. This can result in decreased appetite, which only compounds the problem.

The natural supply of iron with which an infant is born is usually exhausted by 6 months, regardless of a mother's iron intake during pregnancy. At this point, diet becomes an essential source of this mineral. Iron-fortified formulas contain adequate amounts of iron, as does breast milk. After 4 months, as solid foods are introduced, the amount of iron absorbed from breast milk can decrease, so it is particularly important that these solid foods include good sources of iron.

Making the transition

The introduction of more textured foods to your baby's diet should be a gradual one. You can continue to offer some puréed foods and introduce one textured food at a time. There is no need to stop giving all puréed foods at once. Indeed, many infants really enjoy their puréed foods and, by continuing to provide them, you will also have a more precise idea of how much food your child is eating.

Throughout the transition, your child's intake of breast milk or formula will continue to decrease, as solids replace this source of calories. Expect the number of breast feedings to drop to about 4 or 5 per day, while bottles or cups of milk may decrease from 4 to 6 bottles (each 6 to 8 oz [175 to 250 mL]) to about 2 or 3 per day.

Dairy debut

At 11 to 12 months, whole (cow's) milk can replace formula, provided your child's growth and weight gain are good, and he or she is receiving an adequate amount of iron from foods such as infant cereals and meats. (See sidebar for more information about iron.) In fact, to ensure a good supply of dietary iron, you should continue to give your baby iron-fortified infant cereal and/or formula throughout the transition period.

Try substituting formula with whole milk by one-half bottle per day or about one-quarter of total milk intake. You can also mix whole milk with formula or breast milk (half and half) at first, then *gradually* increase amount of whole milk used. A reminder: the calories in whole milk are fewer than in formula – another reason to be sure that intake from solids is adequate.

Don't choke up

At 8 to 12 months, infants are generally able to manage small pieces of soft food without difficulty. Occasionally, however, they can swallow food without mashing it with their tongue or palate, which causes them to choke. The signs of choking can include persistent coughing, gagging, wheezing and sputtering. As alarming as these sounds are, they also mean that the food is not totally blocking the airway – a much more dangerous situation in which the child turns red or blue and makes no sounds at all. (See page 61 for information on infant cardio-pulmonary resuscitation [CPR] – a skill that all parents and caregivers should master.) Where choking sounds are heard, some physicians recommend that you allow the child to cough the food particle out themselves. Other remedies include turning the child upside down to let gravity get food out, or if necessary, giving a few light hits on the back.

Ultimately the best defence against choking is to provide safe foods (see page 62 for a list of foods to avoid) and to monitor your infant constantly during mealtimes.

Choosing starter foods

There are three things to keep in mind when selecting more textured foods to introduce into your baby's diet.

SOFTNESS. Foods should be soft enough to be easily mashed in an infant's mouth. These may include fruits and vegetables (see specific recommendations below), pieces of cheese, meat or fresh bread. To test foods for softness, try mashing them in your own mouth, without using your teeth.

SIZE. Pieces of food should be small enough to eat without choking (see sidebar) – typically no larger than 1/4 to 1/2 inch (5 mm to 1 cm) in size. Pasta (another good starter food) should be cut into similarly short lengths.

VARIETY. Based on the experience you've had feeding your baby puréed or strained foods, you will have already discovered your infant has his or her preferences – vegetables over fruit, for example, or meats over cereals. This is only natural since, as with adults, infants cannot be expected to like all foods equally. Still, it is important to offer your baby a wide variety of textured foods. This helps to build familiarity with a range of tastes and textures. More importantly, it ensures a balanced diet that includes all food groups (see page 77).

Good choices for starter foods include the following.

SOFT FRUITS. These can include ripe *bananas*, *pears* or *peaches* – fresh in season, otherwise canned in juice (avoid the variety packed in heavy syrup, which is excessively sweet and provides a lot of empty calories). Prepare the fruit by slicing then cutting it into pieces approximately 1/4 to 1/2 inch (5 mm to 1 cm) in diameter. Other soft-fruit choices include fresh *mango* (peeled and cut into pieces as above), *seedless grapes* (cut into quarters), *apricots*, *plums*, and *pitted cherries* (cut

Water instead of juice

While fruit juices are often given to young children, they are nutritionally unnecessary for a child whose diet includes fresh fruit. In fact, water is better for quenching thirst and it does not leave residual sugars on the teeth. So get your infant into the water habit early. If you do serve juice, do so only infrequently, and dilute it to half strength.

BETTER BABY FOOD
T I P

To save time, cook fresh vegetables in the microwave oven. In a microwave-safe bowl, add 2 tbsp (25 mL) water to 1 cup (250 mL) vegetables (such as green or wax beans, or broccoli); cover with plastic wrap and cook on High for 3 minutes or until soft. Allow to cool 5 minutes before serving.

into quarters). Many infants enjoy *strawberries* (cut into quarters), but if there is strong history of allergy in your family, you might want to avoid serving them until your baby is at least 1 year old. Other choices include pieces of *papaya* (tasty, but often expensive in colder parts of North America), as well as *melons* (honeydew, cantaloupe) and *avocado*.

VEGETABLES. Cooked until soft, then cooled, vegetables offer a great variety of flavors and textures for your child to enjoy. Good choices include wax or green beans, spinach, carrots, peppers, zucchini and potatoes. Fresh tomatoes (try plum or cherry tomatoes cut in quarters) are also good. Serve vegetables without salt or butter, so your child can enjoy the undisguised taste of each. For best flavor, use fresh produce. Less flavorful but faster to prepare, frozen and (low-sodium) canned vegetables are acceptable substitutes, and they provide comparable nutritional value.

SOFT CHEESES. Try mild or medium Cheddar cheese, grated or thinly sliced and cut into small pieces. (Some infants prefer the stronger cheese, however, so experiment!) Packaged soft cheese products (such as the "Laughing Cow" brand) provide an opportunity to sample different flavors, and are also popular with many young children.

MEATS. These foods are an important source of iron and protein for growing infants and children, but are often the most difficult to get children to eat when starting textures. A good place to start is with chicken, including tender pieces of thigh, leg or breast meat. (Mixing it with some low-salt gravy can help to soften the texture.) Other meat choices include soft beef (from shepherd's pie or stew, for example) or fish without the bones, such as salmon, sole and tuna. Serve canned tuna in its own water or light broth, or mixed with a little mayonnaise. See the meat recipes in this book for suggested preparation methods.

PASTA AND GRAINS. Soft pasta is often an infant favorite. Try "pastina" (child-size pieces of pasta), macaroni, fusili, spaghetti, linguine or penne; serve plain or with butter or a sauce. Be sure to cut long-strand pasta, such as spaghetti or linguine, to prevent your child from gagging or choking. Other grain foods include small pieces of soft bread. Cheerios are also a good choice for their size and consistency.

In all cases, start by giving your infant small amounts of each new food. Keep watch as he or she chews and mashes the food. At this age, you should NEVER leave your infant without supervision while feeding.

Dealing with fussy eaters

When young children are at the stage of trying new foods (as well as their parents' patience!), there will be times when they seem not to be hungry, and refuse their usual favorite foods. This is quite common and should not be a cause for concern. Just as child's growth and weight gain do not always increase smoothly, appetite may also be inconsistent. Also, with all the little things they eat throughout the day, children who refuse a main meal could be getting more food than their parents realize.

Consider, for example, the sample menu shown on page 46. Here a 1-year-old might appear to receive insufficient amounts (bites) of food, yet in fact gets 850 calories – or over 80% of his or her energy needs – from various foods nibbled on throughout the day. (Only 50% of iron needs would be met, however, so you'd eventually need to add iron-rich foods.)

If your child refuses to eat, continue to offer 1 or 2 main items per meal along with milk at the end of the meal. Allow your child to nibble on staple foods such as bread and cheese or pieces of fruit, so that they get some form of nutritious energy.

Try preparing new foods in different ways. For example, you could prepare fish that is cooked with a different sauce, or with different colored vegetables. Show your child that you are enjoying the food that you are offering them. Give them time to eat. Do not hurry your little one's appetite. On the other hand, don't let mealtime go on too long – 20 to 30 minutes is a reasonable limit. Express your delight over the food they do eat. Do not threaten or bribe them with activities or other foods.

BITS AND BITES

Sample menu of a picky (but still well-nourished!) one-year-old eater

Breakfast			Lunch			Supper		
1 oz	cheese	25 g	1 tbsp	tomato pasta sauce	15 mL	Quarter	slice bread	Quarter
Quarter	banana	Quarter	2 tbsp	pasta	25 mL	1	mini yogurt	1
Half	egg	Half	1/4 cup	juice	50 mL		(2 oz [50 g])	
Snack			**Snack**			Quarter	apple	Quarter
6	small bite-size crackers	6	2	arrowroot cookies	2			
Quarter	banana	Quarter	1/4 cup	Cheerios (1 tbsp [15 mL] taken 4 times)	50 mL	2 cups	whole milk (4 servings, each 1/2 cup [125mL], taken throughout the day)	500 mL

Eating out with baby

When having a meal at a restaurant you may find that your infant demonstrates interest in your plate. By all means let the baby try those foods that are soft enough. But try to avoid higher-fat foods (which may not be tolerated well). These include dishes with a rich sauce (such as eggs benedict with Béchamel sauce) or whipped cream on waffles.

Introducing utensils

Between the ages of 8 and 12 months, infants will be able to feed themselves with their hands, but can start to learn to use utensils such as plastic spoons or forks. This will be a messy business, so be prepared. Start by letting your infant watch how you eat with your spoon and fork, then allow him or her to try using utensils with foods such as cereals or yogurt. Chances are there won't be much food that ends up in your child's mouth (not at first, anyway), but eventually he or she will succeed and will feel proud of the accomplishment. Be sure to encourage this new skill enthusiastically.

Teething and tooth care

Teething can begin from as early as 3 months to as late as 10 to 14 months. First teeth cut are usually the incisors (front teeth) which come in around 6 to 8 months. As with most aspects of child development, teething can be more difficult for some

What about fluoride?

If your water supply does not contain fluoride (or contains concentrations of less than 0.3 parts per million), fluoride supplementation may be required when your child's first tooth appears. Why? Fluoride is necessary for proper tooth development. Check with your dentist or pediatrician to see if a supplement is needed. The first trip to the dentist should be at 2 1/2 to 3 1/2 years of age.

BETTER BABY FOOD

T I P

Don't give your child a bottle of juice or milk right before falling asleep. The sugar in either beverage can pool around the teeth and cause decay. Try a bottle of water instead.

infants than others, and can affect their sleeping, general mood and appetite. In many cases, however, teething is used as a catch-all explanation for any of these symptoms when the cause may lie elsewhere. If the symptoms persist, check with your pediatrician or general practitioner. He or she will be able to tell you if teething is the problem (or if there is some other cause) – as well as advise you as to how to deal with teething pain. Remedies may include some pain-relief medication, or using cooled plastic teething rings, biscuits or bagel pieces to teeth on.

What about cleaning your infant's teeth? The time to start is when the teeth first appear. You can begin by using a damp cloth to wipe away plaque. Or you can brush the teeth with a soft baby toothbrush, using a small (less than pea-size) amount of toothpaste once a day. Be sure to wipe or brush the teeth gently, since the gums may be tender, and occasionally you may see some blood. It is a good idea for your child to see you brushing your teeth as well. By 12 months, brushing teeth should be well established, even if the child is not fond of the practice.

Table Food
Q&A

Q. *How do I know when it is safe to feed my child more textures?*

A. You won't really know until you try – with small, soft pieces of food. (Your pediatrician or family doctor can also guide you as to whether your child is ready.) The presence or absence of teeth need not make a difference, since many toothless infants do very well with mashing soft food between their palates (top and bottom of mouth) and tongue.

Q. *What can I do to minimize my child's risk of choking?*

A. Children under the age of 4 years are at the highest risk of choking, and about 75% of choking incidents involve food. But choking can be prevented by ensuring that your child's food is sufficiently soft and is cut into small (no larger than 1/2-inch [1 cm] pieces). Always stay with your child and supervise feeding. Keep infants seated at meal and snack times and do not allow them to run around with food in their mouths. (See page 62 for information on foods that present a danger of choking.)

Q. *What are the signs of allergy to a new food?*

A. Allergic reactions usually manifest themselves in changes to the skin (such as hives or a rash) but may also lead to vomiting or diarrhea. If you suspect an allergy to a certain type of food, eliminate that food from your child's diet for a few weeks. Call your family doctor or pediatrician for advice. (See pages 63 to 67 for more information on allergic reactions to food.)

Q. *When eating in a restaurant, what foods can I safely offer my 10-month-old, who is just starting on textures?*

A. Soft fruits and vegetables or pastas, as well as soft meats, should be fine. Avoid offering foods that are high in fat or sugar. Higher-fat foods tend to remain in the stomach longer, and this sometimes causes stomach upsets.

Q. *Should I give my 8-month-old daughter "junior foods" before offering her table foods?*

A. Commercially prepared "junior foods" are essentially smooth purées with small pieces of food added. They are meant to advance the older infant to more solid textures. Some infants may find it difficult to make the transition from smooth purées to those containing small pieces of solid food. But you do not *need* to use junior foods. Mashing fruits, vegetables or other foods to a thicker consistency is also perfectly acceptable. For example, spaghetti and meat sauce can be puréed in a food processor to a smooth consistency so that pieces of pasta are just visible.

Q. *Should I be switching my child to whole milk or should I offer 2% or 1% milk instead? I am worried about the cholesterol.*

A. Whole milk is generally recommended for infants who are older than 11 or 12 months. You do not have to worry about the cholesterol at this age. The fat in whole milk is an important source of energy for a growing child. However, for infants whose weight is greater than it should be for their length (or height) – or if there is a history of high cholesterol in the family – it may be worth considering 2% milk. Check with your family doctor or pediatrician for advice.

Q. *Should I be giving my 10-month-old infant vitamin or mineral supplements? I want to make sure that he is getting the right amounts.*

A. If your child's diet includes balanced amounts from all the four food groups (see page 77 for more information), then he probably does not need a supplement. However, since many North American children do not get enough iron (even those who are apparently well-fed), you should be sure that he is receiving a sufficient quantity of this mineral through foods such as iron-fortified infant cereal and meat. For example, the recommended daily iron intake for infants between 8 and 12 months can be supplied by 8 tbsp (100 mL) cereal and 4 tbsp (50 mL) meat in a day. (See page 76 for a table of iron requirements.) If you suspect that your child is lacking in one or more specific nutrients, discuss this with your family doctor or pediatrician before offering a supplement. See page 78 for more information about the role of specific vitamins and minerals.

Q. *My child eats much less on some days than on others. Should I be force feeding him or trying to increase the number of snacks offered?*

A. Because a child's growth rate is not always consistent, he may often demonstrate a general lack of interest in food. Other (less frequent) causes can include teething, lack of sleep, snacks too close to mealtime, low iron reserve, or illness. Although poor appetite can be worrying for a parent, don't worry – your child will not starve himself. Chances are he will eat better the next day. If he doesn't, or if his growth or weight gain is below normal, consult with your doctor. Try to avoid tempting your low-appetite child with choice after choice at any given meal. Offer one or two choices and, if they are refused, offer them again at snack time.

Q. *My baby's high chair was given to me by a friend who bought it for her child a number of years ago. I am concerned about it still being safe for my child to use. What are the important features to look for?*

A. A good high chair should have a cushioned, supportive seat; strong, supporting straps; and a foot rest. Other helpful features include wheels (for easy mobility), and a removable tray that can be easily cleaned. (If not cleaned properly, the tray area is a perfect breeding ground for bacteria; wash it thoroughly after each meal, using a clean cloth and soap or a mild detergent, then wipe off with water alone.

Resources

- City of Toronto Department of Public Health "How to prevent choking in children." Fact sheet.

- Gibson, S. A. "Iron intake and iron status of preschool children: associations with breakfast cereals, vitamin C and meat." *Public Health Nutrition* 1999;2:521-528.

- Lozoff, B; Jimenez, E.; Hagen, J; et al. "Poorer behavioural and developmental outcome more than 10 years after treatment for iron deficiency in infancy." *Pediatrics* 2000; 105:E51.

- Martinez, G. A. and Ryan, A. S. "Nutrient intake in the Untied States during the first 12 months of life." *Journal of the American Dietetic Association* 1985; 85:826-830.

- Nutrition Committee, Canadian Paediatric Society. "Meeting the iron needs of infants and young children: an update." *Canadian Medical Association Journal* 1991; 144:1451-1454.

- Oken, E. and Lightdale, J. R. "Updates in pediatric nutrition." *Current Opinion in Pediatrics* 2000; 12:282-290.

- Yeung, G. S. and Zlotkin, S. H. "Efficacy of meat and iron-fortified commercial cereal to prevent iron depletion in cow milk-fed infants 6 to 12 months of age: a randomized controlled trial." *Canadian Journal of Public Health* 2000; 91:263-267.

CHAPTER **5**

The Toddler Years
(12 to 24 months)

SOMEWHERE BETWEEN THE AGES OF 12 AND 24 MONTHS, it suddenly becomes clear that your baby is no longer the helpless creature he or she once was. As speech develops – usually starting with their ability to say "no!" – children are less inclined to accept whatever they are fed. They are able to communicate their preferences of foods more clearly, and to say when they are hungry using words more often than gestures. At this stage, the task of planning meals and feeding your toddler can be quite the challenge. But it can also be fun and rewarding, especially if good eating habits have already been established.

Love that fat!

Fat-phobic parents may hesitate to give their baby whole milk (which contains between 3 and 4% fat). But the added fat and calories are actually good for most young children, which is why whole milk is generally recommended over 2%, 1% or skim milk.

Goodbye formula, hello milk

As long as your child's weight is good, infant formula is usually no longer required after the age of one year. (You can continue breastfeeding, however.) Formulas may still be recommended for those with minimal iron intake or those with poor weight gain. If you are unsure about whether to switch from formula to whole (cow's) milk, ask your family doctor or pediatrician for advice.

If you wish, you can supplement whole milk with iron-fortified formula. (Remember that iron remains an important nutrient at this age, since it is essential for growth.) These have more iron and other minerals than whole milk but, nutritionally speaking, are unnecessary for any child older than 1 year whose diet is varied and includes recommended foods from the various food groups. (See page 77.)

An apple a day?

If your child is able to chew, you may wish to introduce slices of apple. Just keep in mind that an apple is much harder than a banana or peach, so keep a close watch while your child is eating it.

BETTER BABY FOOD
T I P

For a healthier version of french "fries", lightly brushing potato slices or wedges with vegetable oil and bake them until lightly browned.

Bigger
and better

As your child's ability to chew and swallow improves, he or she can manage a greater range of foods.

FRUIT can now be given in larger pieces, although softer varieties – such as bananas, peaches, pears and mangoes – are still recommended. While you can let your child experiment with bite sizes (holding larger pieces or a whole fruit), only do so under close supervision. In cases where a whole fruit could possibly lodge in a small airway (such as grapes or berries), continue to cut the fruit into smaller pieces. Ultimately, let your common sense prevail. Each child develops differently, and you will know what is best suited for your toddler.

VEGETABLES should still be cooked until soft in most cases – although you may wish to try introducing your child to thin slices of fresh cucumber or green peppers. Raw carrots and other hard vegetables can be served if grated. Children also enjoy peas and corn (if only for the exercise in using their fingers), but you should keep a close watch, since it is easy to swallow these vegetables without chewing. Baked potatoes are a good choice, as are (surprisingly) french fries. While higher in fat than baked, french fries still contain many important nutrients and are not the empty-calorie food that many people believe them to be.

MEATS are often more readily accepted as a child gets older and finds them easier to chew – especially when he or she watches the rest of the family eat these foods. Allow your child to sample what the family is having. For more variety of flavor, try preparing meats with herbs and different (mild) spices. (For interesting ideas on how to prepare meat, chicken and fish, try the recipes in this book.)

BETTER BABY FOOD
T I P

Consistent meals and snacks are important for toddlers, as is some form of routine during the day. This includes adequate sleep, play and interactive games.

Timing is *everything*

Wherever possible, try to maintain a reasonable time schedule for meals and snacks. If a child is too tired or hungry, they will not enjoy their meals – and neither will you. Try to ensure that your child gets at least some amount of food around mealtime, and allow the child to have his or her proper rest. Even if you are away from the home, you can provide a light portable meal or more substantial snack (see chart, below). Remember that children like to have a routine, even if they are not in their usual setting. A child's schedule is important, so try to allow for it during the course of your busy day.

BABY FOOD-TO-GO
Portable meals and snacks for your toddler

- French bread (or other fresh bread) with hard or soft cheese spread
- Cereal (such as Cheerios) mixed with crackers or another low-sugar cereal
- Sliced turkey or ham with a fresh roll
- Soup and bread
- Pita bread cut in small pie-shaped pieces, served with vegetable dip (heat pitas for a few seconds in the microwave to make them softer and more appealing)
- Sliced green, yellow or red bell peppers

Nutritious meals in a hurry

As babies grow into toddlers, preparing meals for them often becomes increasingly time-consuming. Here are some helpful and practical tips to fast and nutritious meals.

It is often difficult for many parents to plan their children's meals in advance. But you can still ensure that that they get a nutritious diet by serving a variety of dishes that represent all the main food groups (see page 77), including bread or cereals, vegetables and fruit, milk or milk products, and meat or alternates. For example, a balanced meal could consist of: bread, rice or pasta; a fresh, canned or frozen vegetable; fresh, canned or frozen fruit; and cheese, tofu, or canned tuna with mayonnaise, or leftover chicken or fish sticks. Milk may be given during or after the meal.

Some good "combination meals" include macaroni and cheese, or tuna noodle casserole (which contains grains, fish and milk) – either homemade or store-bought/frozen. For either of these dishes you can add extra cheese, as well as broccoli or some other vegetable for a complete meal.

FAST AND EASY
Quick menus for hungry toddlers

Breakfast 1			Breakfast 2		
1	slice toast with 1/2 tsp (2 mL) butter	1	1/2 cup	iron-rich oatmeal	125 mL
			1/2 cup	whole milk	125 mL
1 oz	cheese, cheddar	25 g	Quarter	orange	Quarter
Quarter	banana	Quarter			
1/2 cup	whole milk	125 mL			
Snack 1			**Snack 2**		
1	oatmeal cookies	1	Half	apple	Half
1/2 cup	whole milk	125 mL	3/4 cup	whole milk	175 mL
Lunch 1			**Lunch 2**		
1/4 cup	spinach soup	50 mL	1/4 cup	green beans with 1/2 tsp (2 mL) butter	50 mL
2	meatballs with mushrooms	2	2	salmon cakes	2
Half	slice bread with 1/2 tsp (2 mL) butter	Half	1/2 cup	whole milk	125 mL
1/2 cup	whole milk	125 mL			
Snack 1			**Snack 2**		
2	unsalted soda crackers	2	Half	banana	Half
1 oz	cheddar cheese	25 g	2	social tea cookies	2
1/4 cup	whole milk	50 mL	1/2 cup	half orange juice, half water	125 mL
Supper 1			**Supper 2**		
1/4 cup	broccoli	50 mL	Quarter	chicken breast	Quarter
1/4 cup	macaroni and cheese	50 mL	1/2 cup	rice with cheese	125 mL
1/2 cup	whole milk	125 mL	1/2 cup	whole milk	125 mL
1/4 cup	strawberries	50 mL	1	slice french bread with with 1/2 tsp (2 mL) butter	1
			1/4 cup	cooked carrots	50 mL
Snack 1			**Snack 2**		
3/4 cup	whole milk	175 mL	1/2 cup	whole milk	125 mL
Calories: 1356	*Protein: 65.2 g*	*Iron: 6.1 mg*	*Calories: 1250*	*Protein: 62 g*	*Iron: 7.0 mg*

BETTER BABY FOOD
T I P

Don't feel that you have to provide a home-cooked meal every day. Time spent hugging and loving your child is important as well.

Shake the salt

Are you worried about the salt (or sodium) content of the food you serve to your children? While a high sodium intake can contribute to high blood pressure in adults, there is no real evidence that it has a similar effect on infants or children, either immediately or later on in life. Still, that doesn't mean you should serve your child very salty foods, or add extra salt to prepared food before they even taste it. And it can't hurt to use less salt when cooking. Just practice moderation. There's nothing wrong with occasionally serving high-sodium processed foods such as deli meats (sliced ham, turkey or chicken), or snack packets of crackers with cheese spread. But try to make sure it's only 1 to 3 times a week.

Soups are also good choices, since you can complement them with bread and cheese, and add tofu for extra protein. Plain cookies – such as arrowroot or digestive – are simple but nutritious desserts. Ice cream served in a small cone is also a welcome treat, and is ideally suited for little hands.

Stocking your pantry

When you have a toddler to feed, be sure to keep some staples on hand (see table, below). Before purchasing packaged foods, read the labels carefully – many contain too much salt (see page 68) and other additives. While commercially prepared meals can be quite nutritious, try to find the time to make a home-cooked meal at least 1 to 3 times a week if at all possible. You'll find it personally satisfying and, as you'll discover with the recipes in this book, easier than you might think.

ESSENTIAL INGREDIENTS
Staple foods to keep on hand

- Milk
- Yogurt
- Eggs
- Cheese
- Bread and low-salt crackers
- Pasta
- Rice
- Cereal (Cheerios, Rice Krispies)
- Frozen peas, beans, other vegetables

- Potatoes, fresh
- Canned fruit
- Canned tuna or salmon
- Frozen fish
- Frozen chicken (breast or thigh)
- Macaroni and cheese (boxed or frozen)
- Canned soup (look for low-sodium variety or dilute with water; add vegetables if desired)

Eating with (and like) grown-ups

Sani-Tray

Feeding trays are often cleaned too quickly and/or not thoroughly enough — especially if the meal has been a prolonged or frustrating one. This can be dangerous, since bacteria like nothing better than a moist area coated with various food residues. So get scrubbing. Use a clean cloth with mild soap, and rinse thoroughly with water.

BETTER BABY FOOD
T I P

If done gradually and with gentle persuasion, you can encourage your child to switch from his or her favorite night time bottle to a "sippy" cup. Just remember that whether it's a bottle or a cup, teeth should always be brushed once it is finished.

Between 12 to 24 months, children continue to build upon the rudimentary self-feeding skills they acquired at the age of 8 to 12 months. In addition, they begin to understand the social aspects of eating with parents and other family members.

Spoons and forks. Developing the skill of using utensils is important for toddlers, since it reinforces their independence. Security and affirmation are extremely important at this stage. So be positive – clapping your hands, smiling and showing approval – as your child gets better at using a spoon and fork. If you are worried about the amount of food actually being eaten, then try starting with spooning food yourself, and let them finish the last two-thirds of the meal. Soup may be more difficult for toddlers to manage on their own, so you may want to guide them with this food. Continue to let them pick up food with their fingers as well.

Toddlers can use their own cutlery, or they may want to try the grown-up version. The special plastic forks and spoons made for children are generally easier to use, however. You can also start serving food on plates (if you have not already done so) instead of putting food on the tray. Toddlers learn quickly that this is where food should be. Try to teach them early on that the plate is not a toy, but meant for food. It can be done! Patience is important.

Taking the cup. By the time your child reaches the toddler stage, you may have already allowed him or her to take sips from your glass. But this is the time to introduce a cup of his or her own. Spill-proof ("sippy") cups are ideal at this age, since they encourage independence and, for bottle-fed children, help to make the transition from bottle to cup.

A family that eats together... Meals are important events to share with your child. Do not use mealtime to get everything done in the kitchen or make phone calls. Try to interact with him or her for at least part of the meal. Allow the child to feed you as well. As you are preparing the food and during the cleanup, talk to your child and explain what you are doing. Describe food that is hot and let them see where hot foods are prepared (the oven or stove). Allow the child to touch hot food, so that they understand what this means. You can teach them to blow on food to let it cool down.

What a mess! As children become more independent in feeding themselves – but before their skills are fully developed – they are capable of creating a substantial mess. So there's no better time to start teaching them the importance of cleaning up. Always clean your child's hands and face after a meal, or let them do this themselves (with a little help from you). Let the child see you clean up the tray and high chair. Have a supply of clean rags on hand to ensure a fresh cloth is used after each meal. You will certainly notice an unpleasant smell from the plastic tray if it is not cleaned properly. The same holds true for bibs. Invest in at least 3 or 4 bibs so that one is always clean and ready to use.

Toddler Years
Q&A

Q. *I don't always have time to prepare homemade meals. Are there nutritious alternatives?*

A. Canned or frozen dinners can be very nutritious, and are good choices when you don't have the time to prepare your own. Read the labels carefully, though, to ensure that they do not contain too much salt or other additives. We recommend that you do try to prepare at least a few of the recipes in this book, however. They're really fast and simple.

Q. *My child has a cold, and I've heard that milk can cause an increase in mucous. Should I avoid milk products?*

A. Simply put, no. There is no research that confirms that milk causes an increase in mucous, so you can safely continue to give your child milk and milk products while he or she is sick. (Milk contains fat, which can adhere to an already mucousy throat and cause a sensation, albeit a false one, of increased mucous.) The important thing to consider is that milk is an essential source of Vitamin D and calcium (both important for bone growth), as well as protein and energy.

Q. *My child refuses to eat vegetables. What can I do?*

A. While many children dislike one or two vegetables, it is unusual to hate them all. The important thing is that you don't become discouraged if your child refuses a vegetable once. Introduce it again using a different preparation method, or at a different temperature and with a different food. Experiment with sauces or dressings (in small amounts) to enhance flavor. Focus on those vegetables that are popular with most children, such as corn, peas, carrots, beans and sweet potatoes. Soups are another good way to get your child to eat vegetables. (See the many soup recipes in this book for ideas.)

Q. *How often should my daughter have snacks? I usually give her Cheerios and digestive cookies because they're so convenient. What other healthy snacks can you suggest?*

A. Snacks are a very important part of your child's diet, and should be offered at least 2 to 3 times a day. This will prevent her from getting too hungry and tired before mealtime, and will allow you some flexibility in your schedule. For an alternative to your current snacks, try fresh fruit, cut into small bite-size pieces, or vegetables such as slices of green or red bell peppers; these can be kept in a plastic bag and enjoyed at any time. Other nutritious snacks include grated cheese, pieces of a bagel, pita or other kinds of bread, low-salt crackers, and treats such as homemade cookies. (See pages 223 to 246 for more snack ideas.)

Q. *My husband tends to feed our daughter more quickly than I do, with result that she eats less, and anticipates playtime less patiently. I often want to feed her myself, because I know that she will feed better for me, but realize that my husband has to feed her as well. What can we do to remedy this?*

A. It is important for both of you to be consistent in your approach to feeding. Have your husband eat with your child, preferably for the same amount of time that you do. Make sure you both interact with your child at mealtimes, and that you are not using that time to read the paper, answer phone calls or read the mail. Above all, discuss the importance of consistency with your husband, and allow some time for change to take place. But remember also that there are many reasons why a child may be eating less (such as teething, fatigue or illness).

Q. *I have heard that some children tolerate goat's milk better than cow's milk. Is this true?*

A. No. Not if they have an allergy to cow's milk. Children with an allergy to cow's milk protein should not be given goat's milk as an alternative, since they will most likely react to the protein in goat's milk as well. Other claims of better tolerance to goat's milk are not supported by any research. Goat's milk is similar to cow's milk in that it is a good source of many important nutrients, including calcium and vitamin D. One difference between the two is in the types of protein each contains. Goat's milk may be deficient in folic acid (which is important for the production of red blood cells). If you choose goat's milk, make sure that it has folic acid added.

Q. *We drink soda pop in our house, and my 18-month-old son keeps asking to try some. Is it okay to give him a few sips?*

A. Soda pop provides little in the way of beneficial nutrients except for calories and, in some cases, a bit of vitamin C. In addition, many of these drinks contain significant amounts of caffeine. As such, they are not really suitable for toddlers. Of course, a few sips here or there will not damage his health. A better alternative is to mix 1 part fruit juice with 3 parts unflavored sparkling water (such as Perrier. This is a refreshing, tasty drink that is good for your toddler – and the whole family.

Resources

- Bellioni-Businco, B.; Paganelli, R.; Lucotti, P.; Giampietro, P; Perborn, H; and Businco, L. "Allerginicity of goat's milk in children with cow's milk allergy." *Journal of Allergy and Clinical Immunology* 1999; 103:1191.

- Dennison, B. A. "Fruit juice consumption by infants and children: a review." *Journal of the American College of Nutrition* 1996; 15:4S-11S.

- Dennison, B.A.; Rockwell, H. L.; and Baker, S. L. "Fruit and vegetable intake in young children." *Journal of the American College of Nutrition* 1998; 17:371-378.

- Ellison, R. C.; Singer, M. R.; Moore, L. L.; et al. "Current caffeine intake of young children: amount and sources." *Journal of the American Dietetic Association* 1995; 95:802-804.

- Koivisto Hursti, U. K. "Factors influencing children's food choice. *Annals of Medicine* 1999; 31:26-32.

- Picciano, M. F.; Smiciklas-Wright, H.; Birch, L. L.; et al. "Nutritional guidance is needed during dietary transition in early childhood." *Pediatrics* 2000; 106:109-114.

- Roberts, S. B. and Heyman, M. B. "Micronutrient shortfalls in young children's diets: common, and owing to inadequate intakes both at home and at child care centers." *Nutrition Reviews* 2000; 58:27-29.

- Young, B. and Drewett, R. "Eating behaviour and its variability in 1-year-old children." *Appetite* 2000; 35:171-177.

CHAPTER **6**

Adverse Reactions to Food

Many foods that are safe for adults can be dangerous for young children. For example, a food's consistency may be such that it is hard to chew and/or swallow, thereby presenting a choking hazard. A food may be contaminated with bacteria, or it may contain compounds that cause an allergic reaction. Foods may cause digestive problems such as diarrhea or constipation. In each of these cases, it is important that parents understand the risks and remedies involved.

CPR certified?

If your child, or someone else's child, were to choke in your presence, would you know how to handle the situation? With training in infant cardio-pulmonary resuscitation (CPR) you would be prepared. Infant CPR training can be organized through your local community center or the Red Cross. (Keep in mind that infant CPR is very different from adult CPR.) You may be able to get someone qualified to come to your home, where they can teach a group of friends and family.

Choking hazards

Anyone who has been around infants knows that they love to put things in their mouths. This makes them very susceptible to choking. Also, when eating, some infants swallow food without mashing it with their tongue or palate, which causes them to gag or to choke. Parents need to do all they can to minimize the risk of choking for their children.

Children should always be supervised while eating. Do not allow toddlers to walk or run with food in their mouths. Eating in the car is also considered unsafe for young children: If they choke in the car, you may not be able to pull over to the curb safely to help them. In addition, unexpected motion in a car (such as a sudden stop) can cause choking.

For infants, a "propped bottle" (that is, where no one is holding the bottle) is potentially hazardous, since the flow of milk can exceed the infant's ability to drink it, thereby causing him or her to choke.

Many foods are considered unsafe for toddlers because of their shape. These include hard, sticky foods that have the potential to block their small airways. Some of these foods are listed in the table below.

HARD TO SWALLOW
Foods to avoid for children under 4 years old

Popcorn	Cough drops	Sunflower seeds	Whole carrots
Hard candies	Raisins (whole)	Fish with bones	Gum
Peanuts/nuts	Snacks with toothpicks/skewers		

Post this list on your refrigerator for all family members and friends to read.

Food-borne illness

Infants are at an increased risk of "food poisoning" because of their immature digestive and immune systems. Food-borne illnesses are caused by eating foods contaminated with bacteria, viruses, parasites, or bacterial or chemical toxins. Parents can help minimize the risk of these illnesses by taking the following precautions:

• Hot food should be kept hot and cold food should be kept cold. Bacteria multiply quickly under the warm temperatures in between.

• Make sure that all foods of animal origin are cooked well. This includes beef, fish, pork, chicken and eggs.

• Wash hands thoroughly to prevent cross-contamination when preparing food. Raw foods should not come in contact with hands that have been dealing with cooked foods and vice versa.

• Keep work surfaces and utensils clean. Wash surfaces and utensils thoroughly with soap and water when in contact with raw foods.

• Store foods properly at the correct temperature. Refrigerate leftovers as soon as possible.

• Thaw frozen foods in the refrigerator or under cold running water. Do not thaw foods on the counter at room temperature.

• Read the "best before" date when purchasing items. Do not buy cracked, dirty or unrefrigerated eggs. Do not purchase canned foods that are dented or if the top of the can is bulging.

• Honey should not be offered to infants less than 12 months old. This includes all food products that contain honey as an ingredient. Honey may contain spores of the bacterium *Clostridium botulinum*, which can cause infant botulism.

Food
allergies

BETTER BABY FOOD

T I P

Breastfeeding can help to protect against certain allergies. Genetic factors may also play a role in determining which children are at greater risk for developing allergies.

Food allergy or "hypersensitivity" is defined as an immune-system response to a food protein that the body identifies as foreign. As such, it is different from a food *intolerance* (such as lactose intolerance), which is an adverse reaction to a food that results in symptoms, but is not caused by a reaction of the immune system.

Children under 5 years are especially susceptible to food allergies because of their immature digestive system. The lining in the digestive tract is very permeable or "leaky" in the first months of life, which allows allergens to pass into the bloodstream and come in contact with the cells of the immune system.

As the digestive system matures over the first 3 to 4 years of life, it is able to exclude these larger, potentially allergenic molecules. It is in the first year, however, that most sensitization to food allergy occurs. If potentially allergenic foods can

Extreme reaction

Anaphylaxis is an intense, immediate allergic response. Symptoms can include hives, swelling around the mouth and face, itching, difficulty breathing, nausea and diarrhea. Severe cases can lead to anaphylactic shock or even death. Anaphylactic symptoms usually occur within minutes of food ingestion, but can occur up to 1 or 2 hours later. Parents of children with anaphylactic reactions to foods must carry an injection containing epinephrine (for example, Epipen®) at all times. A prescription can be obtained through your physician, pediatrician or immunologist.

BETTER BABY FOOD
T I P

You should not immediately eliminate a food from your child's diet because you suspect he or she is allergic to it. This can result in an unbalanced diet, leading to poor weight gain, as well as possible vitamin or mineral deficiencies. Suspected food allergies should be confirmed before the food is eliminated.

be avoided avoided during this time, a food allergy may be avoided or not be as severe.

Allergic reactions can manifest themselves in a number of ways, including:

Systemic: anaphylaxis; failure to gain appropriate weight

Digestive: vomiting; abdominal pain; diarrhea; malabsorption of nutrients

Respiratory: runny nose; nasal congestion; difficulty breathing; wheezing

Skin: rash, hives, eczema

Diagnosing
food allergies

If you suspect that your child has a food allergy (or if you have a strong family history of allergies), it is important that you have him or her tested. There are several methods for doing this.

Double-blind placebo/controlled-food challenge. In this test, the offending allergen or a placebo (blank/dummy) capsule is given orally and neither the patient nor the clinician knows which is which. The patient's reaction and symptoms are then monitored by the clinician.

Elimination diet. With this method, allergenic foods are eliminated from the diet for a 2-week period and are then slowly reintroduced to try and identify which foods are causing symptoms. This diet should be followed under medical supervision. The testing period should not exceed 2 weeks, since nutritional deficiencies may result.

Skin test. Also known as "prick tests", these are widely used to diagnose food allergy. A small amount of an allergen is introduced to the skin by pricking the skin with a small needle. The skin is then monitored for a reaction. Skin tests are not 100% accurate, and false positives (a reaction in the absence of true allergy) may occur. These tests are unreliable for infants and are not used in such cases.

Types of
food allergies

While any number of foods can cause allergic reactions, there are several that have proven to be more widespread than others.

Milk allergy. Cow's milk allergy occurs in about 2 or 3 of every 100 infants – although most grow out of it by the time they are 3 years old. Infants at higher risk for developing milk allergy include those cases where one or both parents (or a sibling) had milk allergy as an infant. Symptoms of milk allergy include vomiting, diarrhea and insufficient weight gain. Blood in the stools, colic, skin or chest symptoms may also occur. Blood loss secondary to cow's milk allergy may also cause iron deficiency anemia in children. If your child has been diagnosed by a physician with cow's milk allergy, it is important that you obtain dietary counseling to ensure the proper nutrients are provided, especially calcium and vitamin D – both of which are normally supplied by cow's milk and are needed for the development of strong bones and teeth.

WHERE'S THE MILK?

Milk ingredients are not always clearly indicated as such on food labels. If you see any of the following words on a label, it means the food contains milk protein.

milk	cheese	cream	casein
condensed milk	cottage cheese	cream cheese	sodium caseinate
evaporated milk	sour cream	quark®	potassium caseinate
milk powder	yogurt	ice cream	whey
butter	buttermilk	sherbet	lactoglobulin
milk solids	curd	feta/ricotta	lactose

Source: Vickerstaff-Joneja, J. Managing Food Allergy and Intolerance: A Practical Guide. *1995*

Tips for egg-free baking

1. Where egg is used as a leavening agent: For each egg, substitute 1 tbsp egg-free baking powder + 2 tbsp liquid OR 2 tbsp flour + 1/2 tbsp (7 mL) egg-free baking powder + 2 tbsp (15 mL) liquid. The liquid can be anything that is appropriate for the recipe (such as water, vinegar, fruit juice, broth). Some recipes call for only one egg and a large proportion of baking powder – for example, 2 tsp (10 mL) baking powder or 1 1/2 tsp (7 mL) baking soda. Try these recipes without the egg and add 1 tbsp (15 mL) vinegar instead.

2. Where egg is used as a binder: For each egg, substitute 1/3 cup (75 mL) water combined with 3 to 4 tsp (15 to 20 mL) brown flax seeds; bring to a boil over high heat, then simmer on low heat for 5 to 7 minutes until a slightly thickened gel begins to form; strain liquid and use the gel in recipe. Other substitutes include 1/3 cup (75 mL) water + 1 tbsp (15 mL) arrowroot powder + 2 tsp (10 mL) guar gum OR 2 oz (50 g) tofu.

3. Where egg is used as a liquid: For each egg, substitute 1/3 cup (75 mL) apple juice OR 4 tbsp (60 mL) puréed apricot OR 1 tbsp (15 mL) vinegar.

Egg allergy. Because this type of allergy is common in young children, most authorities recommend that delaying the introduction of egg yolk until an infant is 6 months old. The introduction of egg whites, where most of the protein is found, should be delayed until an infant is at least 12 months old.

For infants who have a confirmed allergy to eggs, avoiding whole eggs is fairly easy. But because eggs are so widely as an ingredient, it is often much harder to avoid foods that may contain eggs. For example, some common foods that contain eggs include custards, egg nog, caesar salad, cakes, cookies, pies, pancakes, waffles and battered foods. Eggs may also be used in consommé soup and soft drinks (such as root beer), where it is used as a clarifier. Egg Beaters®, while sold as an egg substitute, is not egg-free and should not be consumed by infants or toddlers with an egg allergy.

Some vaccinations also contain egg protein. Your physician will be able to give you more information if you are concerned about egg allergy and vaccines.

- -

EGG INDICATORS
If you see any of the following words on a food label, it contains egg protein.

albumin	mayonnaise
egg	egg powder
baking powder	egg powder
ovalbumin	ovoglobulin
egg white	egg protein
ovomucin	ovomucoid
egg yolk	frozen egg
ovovitellin	pasteurized egg
globulin	simplesse®
livetin	vitellin

Source (table above and sidebar at left): Source: Vickerstaff-Joneja, J. Managing Food Allergy and Intolerance: A Practical Guide. 1995

- -

Allergen-Free Baking Powder

While some types of baking powder (such as Magic brand) are egg-free, others are not. To make a substitute, combine 1 part baking soda with 2 parts cream of tartar and 1 part cornstarch. Mix well and store in airtight container.

Source: Managing Food Allergy and Intolerance. A Practical Guide Vickerstaff

BETTER BABY FOOD
T I P

Some children with an allergy to raw eggs are able to tolerate cooked eggs. This is because heat breaks down some – but not all – of the egg proteins.

Peanut allergy. Unlike milk and egg allergies, a peanut allergy generally persists beyond childhood. This type of allergy is common, as well as being one of the most severe – often the cause of anaphylactic shock. While a peanut allergy does not necessarily extend to all nuts, a child who has had a previous anaphylactic reaction to peanuts should avoid all nuts to be safe. Pure peanut oil should also be avoided, since, although theoretically free of peanut proteins, may nevertheless contain trace amounts. Peanut oil is widely used in many restaurants (particularly Thai and Chinese), so you may wish to avoid these restaurants altogether. Also, be sure to read labels carefully for foods that "may contain" peanuts. These foods should not be consumed by an infant or toddler with a peanut allergy.

Wheat allergy. While not common, grain allergies do occur, with wheat as the most likely cause. This allergy is an adverse reaction to the protein component of wheat. It is different from *celiac disease*, in which affected patients cannot tolerate *gluten* (a protein found in many grains, including wheat, oats, rye and barley). Celiac disease requires significant lifelong dietary changes, beyond eliminating wheat from the diet.

Wheat is found in many foods, including breads, cereals, pastas, cakes, luncheon meats and sausage – virtually anything that contains wheat flour. Because wheat flour is often fortified with vitamins such as riboflavin, thiamin, niacin and iron (as it is in the U.S. and Canada, for example), the elimination of wheat from an allergic child's diet can result in a nutrient deficiency unless replaced by other foods, including alternate flours such as rye, corn, or rice. It is important that the parent of any child with a confirmed allergy to wheat speak to a registered dietitian about the specific dietary changes that are involved.

Food
additives

While their effects are uncertain, food additives are often blamed for causing changes in children's behavior. For example, many parents claim they cause conditions such as attention deficit disorder. Food additives include artificial food colorings and flavors, preservatives (such as sulfur dioxide, butylated hydroxytoluene [BHT] and butylated hydroxyanisole [BHA]), nitrates and nitrites, as well as artificial sweeteners. Many scientific studies have been conducted over the years to assess the effects of additives on children. While some have found that certain additives have an affect on behavior, not all reached the same conclusion.

For parents who believe that eliminating additives will improve a child's behavior, then this should be done through objective evaluation, under the supervision of a family doctor. This will require taking objective measurements of their child's behavior before the new diet is started, and several days after it is started. Objective measures may include recording the exact amount of time (in minutes or hours) that certain behaviors are observed over a defined period of days.

Dealing with
diarrhea

The primary causes of diarrhea are infection. The condition is defined as when infants or children have excessive stool – that is, greater than 20 to 50 mL per kg of body weight per day or 1 to 2 cups (250 to 500 mL) per day for a 1 year old) — and where the output is changed from its normal consistency. (Keep in mind that infants' stools can vary in frequency and consistency from day to day, and from infant to infant.) Typically, this means the stool has more water than usual and is more frequent.

Infants younger than 6 to 8 months are especially vulnerable to the consequences of diarrhea. This is because of the risk of dehydration, due to the potential large fluid losses. A family doctor should always be consulted when diarrhea lasts greater than 24 hours in young infants.

The consistency of diarrhea can be watery, mucousy or oily. Each provides an indication as to the cause of the diarrhea.

Watery diarrhea usually occurs as a result of intolerance to carbohydrate (sugar), often lactose or sorbitol. Intolerance to lactose (found in cow's milk) can occur temporarily following a viral infection that affects the gut lining, decreasing the amount of the enzyme lactase. (Lactase is needed to break down lactose.) Sorbitol is found in some juices (non-citrus varieties, such as apple, pear and prune juices) which, if ingested in large amounts, can also cause watery diarrhea.

Overstimulated?

Sugar and chocolate may be considered additives, and many parents claim these also cause an increase in hyperactivity in their children. Caffeine, a known stimulant found in varying amounts in chocolate, has a metabolic reason for its effects on increasing activity. There is no scientific evidence that sugar causes hyperactivity or disruptive behavior in children.

Mucousy stools can be caused by a viral or bacterial infection. It may indicate inflammation of the colon. Sometimes a change in formula (to a more predigested formula, for example) can also result in more mucousy stool, although volume is not usually increased. With a viral infection, stools increase in volume.

Oily stools are a sign that fats are not being digested properly. Causes of this can include disorders of the pancreas, intolerance of gluten (protein found in bread and other cereals). Stools may be formed, or loose, and are usually excessive and foul-smelling.

Other causes of diarrhea include milk-protein sensitivity, which is the most common milk-related illness among infants. Diarrhea (and vomiting) can occur as soon as milk protein is ingested, with a typical onset being anywhere between 2 days and 4 months of age. For more information on milk allergies, see pages 22 to 23, and 65.

Soothing sore bums

Diaper rash is a common after effect of diarrhea. If the rash is severe, try Ihle's paste, which contains corn starch and zinc, or another cream with zinc (preferably with a zinc content of more than 10%), and use it liberally with each diaper change. When wiping buttocks, use only tissue and water. Cotton balls or make-up-remover pads are also good. Keep a plastic container of water in a drawer or near change table area for convenience. The astringent in commercial diaper wipes (even those that are scent-free) can irritate sensitive infant skin, so avoid using these when your child has a rash.

BETTER BABY FOOD

TIP

Not always constipated. Keep in mind that stooling patterns in young children can vary from day to day. Less frequent stooling may not necessarily mean they are constipated.

Treatment

The first step in treating diarrhea is to replace the fluid and electrolytes (salts) that have been lost. If the diarrhea lasts for longer than a day (depending on the age of the infant), rehydration solutions (such as Pedialyte®) may be used for a period of 24 hours. After this, a normal diet can be resumed. (Note: if vomiting was associated with the diarrhea, then refeeding should begin as soon as vomiting has stopped.) Your doctor will guide you on the type, volume and duration of rehydration solution to give your child. Remember to ask how long the solution is to be used for, and when a full diet can be reintroduced.

Child
constipation

Constipation is defined as a reduced water content in the stool and is caused by insufficient water in the colon. It is one of the most common disorders in western society, affecting children and adults alike. Despite numerous studies, the dietary factors leading to constipation remain unclear. One study concluded that insufficient calorie and nutrient intake, as well as a decrease in body weight, were associated with constipation. Cow's milk allergy may cause constipation and reflux, but this cause is rare.

Symptoms

How do you know if your child is constipated? Stools may appear like small pellets, or they may be in the form of one very large round ball. They are usually difficult for your child to pass. Mucus may also appear in the stool, and it may be slightly blood-streaked. This is not normally a cause for concern. The mucus is from the lining of the intestine and the blood may represent a small tear in the lining. If the bleeding persists or appears heavier than a slight streak, then contact your doctor.

There are medical causes for chronic constipation (other than dietary), and these will be investigated if your doctor has reason for concern. In most cases, however, diet is the source of the problem.

Treatment

Providing an adequate supply of fluids is essential to the treatment of constipation. If your house is kept very warm in the winter, or is hot in the summer months, then extra fluid must be provided. Daily fluid intake (including all sources of fluid) should be approximately 4 to 6 cups (1 to 1.5 L).

If your child is on solids, offer a varied diet, with plenty of fresh fruits and vegetables. Offer cereals daily, and try a few teaspoons of bran cereal mixed in with oatmeal or infant cereal for children older than 12 to 18 months.

If your child shows signs of difficulty with a bowel movement – straining or grunting, for example, or becoming red in the face and crying – you can provide some relief by laying the infant on the change area and pull his or legs up, then massaging the stomach gently.

If constipation cannot be relieved through dietary measures, or if it is very severe, then *lactulose* (an undigestable sugar) may be prescribed by your family doctor or pediatrician. Only a small amount of the lactulose is required to promote fecal movement and softer stools. Glycerin suppositories may also be prescribed.

Iron and constipation

Iron-fortified formulas have not been proven to cause constipation, and iron given as a supplement may change the color of stool but does not cause constipation. If your child requires an iron supplement, check with your doctor to see how long it is prescribed for. Ensure that your child's diet provides an adequate supply of iron once the supplement is discontinued.

Resources

JOURNALS

- Baker, S. S.; Liptak, G. S.; Colletti, R. B.; et al. "Constipation in infants and children: evaluation and treatment." *Journal of Pediatric Gastroenterology and Nutrition* 1999; 29:612-626.

- Hyams, J. S.; Etienne, N. L.; Leichtner, A. M.; and Theuer, R. C. "Carbohydrate malabsorption following fruit juice ingestion in young children." *Pediatrics* 1988; 82:64-68.

- Hyams, J. S.; Treem, W. R.; Etienne, N. L.; et al. "Effect of infant formulas on stool characteristics of young infants." *Pediatrics* 1995; 95:50-54

- Nutrition Committee, Canadian Paediatric Society. "Oral rehydration therapy and early refeeding in the management of childhood gastroenteritis." *Canadian Journal of Paediatrics* 1994;1:160-164.

- Pollock, I. and Warner, J. O. "Effect of artificial food colours on childhood behaviour." *Archives of Disease in Childhood* 1990; 65:74-77.

- Skinner, J. D.; Carruth, B. R.; Moran, J. III; et al. "Fruit juice is not related to children's growth." *Pediatrics* 2000; 105(3):e38-44.

- Wilson, N. and Scott, A. "A double-blind assessment of additive intolerance in children using a 12 day challenge period at home." *Clinical and Experimental Allergy* 1989; 19:267-272.

- Wolraich, M. L.; Lindgren, S. D.; Stumbo, P. J.; et al. "Effects of diets high in sucrose or aspartame on the behavior and cognitive performance of children." *New England Journal of Medicine* 1994; 330:301-307.

WEB SITES

- Dietitians of Canada   www.dietitians.ca

- American Dietetic Association   www.eatright.org

- Food Allergy Network   www.foodallergy.org

- Specialty Food Shop   www.specialtyfoodshop.com
  or call 1-800-SFS-7976 or 416-977-4360. Purchase wheat free, milk free, egg free products. Catalogue available. Dietitians available to answer questions. Associated with the Hospital for Sick Children.

CHAPTER 7

Nutrition Facts

It goes without saying (particularly in a book like this one) that good nutrition is essential to the health of a child. And while today's parents are generally more diet-conscious than any generation before them, the task of sorting out all the information now available about nutrition can be a little overwhelming. Our advice to worried parents? Relax. A balance of good, nutritious foods and regular exercise is generally all your child needs. It is only in a small number of circumstances – for example, in cases of iron-deficiency or where a strict vegetarian diet is being followed – that special dietary measures may be required. In this chapter, we'll look at some of these issues, as well as the basic components of a healthy, balanced diet.

Food fundamentals

Food provides the essential elements that the body requires for growth and metabolism. These include carbohydrates, proteins, fats, minerals and vitamins.

Carbohydrates are sugars of various types that provide the body with energy. Common sources include breads and cereals, as well as fruits and vegetables.

Proteins are complex structures of different amino acids that the body uses to build tissue as well as other proteins that carry out specific functions within the body, such as fighting infections. Examples of protein foods include meat and fish.

Fats are a good source of energy. By weight, fat has more than double the calories found in either carbohydrates or proteins. They also provide essential fatty acids that are important for a variety of bodily functions. Fat is found in dairy products, meats, fish and oils.

Minerals and **vitamins** are essential to the proper functioning of the body's metabolism. This is especially true when the body is growing as quickly – as it does in infancy and childhood – and establishes a foundation for a healthy adult life.

Dairy-free dilemma

Children who can't drink milk because of a milk protein allergy or lactose intolerance may require a supplement of calcium and vitamin D. Soy beverages, which are often given to replace cow's milk, may not be adequate to prevent the development of rickets unless they are fortified with supplemental vitamin D and calcium. Be sure to check any milk-free substitutes to ensure that they contain sufficient amounts of these essential nutrients. If you are unsure, check with your doctor or dietitian. Keep in mind, too, that dairy-free beverages may also contain less fat (and energy) than cow's milk.

Vitamins and minerals to watch

While all vitamins and many minerals are important for the growing needs of a healthy child, there are some that deserve special attention, since they may be deficient in a poorly balanced North American diet. For the list of other vitamins and minerals and their role in metabolism, see page 78.

Calcium and vitamin D are essential for growth and maintenance of healthy bones and teeth. If a child does not receive adequate amounts of these nutrients daily, then the deficiency can lead to rickets – a condition in which the bones soften, making them more susceptible to breakage or to a bowing of the legs when the child learns to walk. Rickets can occur in exclusively breast-fed infants who are not provided with a vitamin D supplement (see page 13).

Good dietary sources of calcium and vitamin D include milk and cheese. Sunshine is also a good source of vitamin D (which is produced when skin absorbs the sun rays). It doesn't take much – only 15 to 20 minutes per day is necessary.

HOW MUCH CALCIUM?
Recommended daily calcium intakes

Age	RDA (US)*	RNI (Canada)*	DRI (US/Can)*
0 to 6 months	400 mg	250 mg (0 to 4 months)	210 mg
6 months to 1 year	600 mg	400 mg (5 to 12 months)	270 mg
1 to 2 years	800 mg	500 mg (1 year)	500 mg
2 to 3 years	800 mg	550 mg (2 to 3 years)	500 mg

HOW MUCH VITAMIN D?
Recommended daily vitamin D intakes

Age	RDA (US)*	RNI (Canada)*	DRI (US/Can)*
0 to 6 months	7.5 µg**	10 µg (0 to 4 months)	5 µg
6 to 12 months	10 µg	10 µg (5 to 12 months)	5 µg
1 to 3 years	10 µg	15 µg (2 to 3 years)	5 µg

* Prior to 1997, the US and Canada used different standards for recommended intakes of energy and nutrients – respectively, the RDA (Recommended Dietary Allowances) and RNI (Recommended Nutrient Intakes). Since then, a new standard, the DRI (Dietary Reference Intakes), has been gradually introduced to provide a single reference for Americans and Canadians. For certain nutrients, 1989 RDA figures have been replaced by DRIs.
** 1 µg = 1 microgram   (1 mg = 1 milligram)

Iron is a very important nutrient for growing children. It is part of a blood component called hemoglobin, which is necessary for the transport, storage and use of oxygen throughout the body. All babies are born with a supply of iron, which takes them through the first 4 to 6 months of life. After that, iron must be obtained through the diet.

For infants and young children, iron-fortified infant cereals are the primary source of iron from solid foods. Meats are also an excellent source of iron (see Tip). Iron is also supplied by spinach, peas and dark green vegetables – although the type of iron found in these foods is not as readily absorbed as that found in meats.

Iron from meats is called *heme* iron; the type found in vegetables and grains is called *non-heme* iron. This distinction is generally not provided on food labels, but it is an important one to remember, since heme iron is absorbed 2 to 3 times better than the non-heme form.

Children who do not obtain an adequate supply of iron in their diet run the risk of developing *iron-deficiency anemia,* a condition that arises when hemoglobin falls below normal levels. A child with this condition is typically pale, tires easily and has a lower tolerance for exercise. Other symptoms include irritability and decreased appetite.

Iron-deficiency anemia is most common worldwide among infants and children from 6 months to 3 years of age – a period during which the child's natural stores of iron have been exhausted (and must be obtained through diet), and during which the child requires substantial amounts of iron to fuel his or her rapid growth. Typically, the danger period is most acute between the ages of 12 to 18 months, when children make the transition from iron-fortified foods (such as formula and infant rice cereal) to solids that, while otherwise nutritious, may contain less iron. It is also at this age that children switch to cow's milk, which can displace iron-rich foods and has the effect of reducing iron absorption from other foods. (This effect can be minimized by restricting milk intake to between meals.)

BETTER BABY FOOD
T I P

While meats are a good source of iron, they may not appeal to younger children, who may also find these foods hard to chew. Good choices include moist pieces of chicken and beef that have been prepared with a variety of herbs and flavors. Meatballs are always a favorite. (See pages 174, 175 and 201 for recipes.).

BETTER BABY FOOD
T I P

To enhance iron absorption from non-heme sources such as vegetables and grains, serve these foods with other foods that are high in vitamin C, such as oranges or strawberries.

Treatment of iron deficiency anemia usually requires an oral supplement of iron. If the response to this treatment is poor (that is, if hemoglobin levels do not return to normal), other causes of iron deficiency must be ruled out. Once hemoglobin levels return to normal, then iron supplementation can be discontinued, provided the diet supplies an adequate amount. (See list, below.)

PUMPING IRON
Food sources rich in iron

Food	Serving size	Iron (mg)
Liver	1.75 oz (45 g)	9.0
Cream of wheat	3/4 cup (175 mL)	9.0
Infant cereal	8 tbsp (120 mL)	6.7
Infant formula, fortified	8 oz (250 mL)	5.0
Spinach, cooked	1/2 cup (125 mL)	3.2
Potato, baked, skin on	6.5 oz (190 g)	2.75
Beans, navy, canned	1/2 cup (125 mL)	2.42
Beef, lean broiled	3.5 oz (100 g)	2.35
Raisins, seedless	2/3 cup (150 mL)	2.08
Avocado	1 medium	2.04
Rice, white, enriched	1 cup (250 mL)	1.8
Prune juice	1/2 cup (125 mL)	1.51
Chicken, light/dark, no skin	3.5 oz (100 g)	1.21
Halibut	3 oz (75 g)	0.91
Broccoli, cooked	1/2 cup (125 mL)	0.89
Whole wheat bread	1 slice	0.86
Strained infant meat	4 tbsp (60 mL)	0.78
White bread	1 slice	0.68
Apricots, raw	3 medium	0.58

HOW MUCH IRON?
Recommended daily iron intakes

Age	RDA (US)	RNI (Canada)
0 to 6 months	6 mg	0.3 mg
6 months to 1 year	10 mg	7 mg
1 to 3 years	10 mg	6 mg

Vitamin C is essential for healing. It is also helpful in enhancing iron absorption and, many believe, in fighting colds (although there is no definitive clinical evidence to support this). A diet that includes fresh fruits containing large amounts of vitamin C – such as mangoes, oranges and strawberries – will help to ensure that your child is getting enough. Fruit juices, such as orange and apple juice, also contain vitamin C, but are less nutritious than fresh fruit. Excess amounts of vitamin C, as with most vitamins, can be dangerous, and can actually lead to a deficiency when discontinued. This is called rebound scurvy, which can cause bleeding gums and lips.

How much vitamin C?
Recommended daily vitamin C intakes

Age	RDA (US)*	RNI (Canada)*	DRI (US/Can)*
0 to 6 months	30 mg	20 mg (0 to 4 months)	40 mg
6 months to 1 year	35 mg	20 mg (5 to 12 months)	50 mg
1 to 3 years	40 mg	20 mg (2 to 3 years)	15 mg

* Prior to 1997, the US and Canada used different standards for recommended intakes of energy and nutrients – respectively, the RDA (Recommended Dietary Allowances) and RNI (Recommended Nutrient Intakes). Since then, a new standard, the DRI (Dietary Reference Intakes), has been gradually introduced to provide a single reference for Americans and Canadians. For certain nutrients, 1989 RDA figures have been replaced by DRIs.

The fab four food groups

BETTER BABY FOOD

T I P

While excessive doses of vitamins have become popular with some adults, they should never be given to children. Check with your pediatrician, family doctor, dietitian or pharmacist to learn what amounts are safe for your child.

While many foods are important sources of nutrients, there is no single food that provides everything you need for a healthy diet. That's why it's important to enjoy a balanced diet that includes all four food groups.

Breads and cereals are an essential source of carbohydrates, vitamins and minerals, and provide fiber as well.

Fruits and vegetables provide another variety of carbohydrates, vitamins (particularly vitamin C) and minerals, as well as fiber.

Meat and alternates are an important source of proteins, fats, vitamins and minerals (particularly iron).

THE ABCs OF VITAMINS AND MINERALS
Essential nutrients at a glance

Vitamin/mineral	Type	Assists in	Sources
Vitamin A (from beta-carotene)	Fat-soluble	Vision, growth, bone development, healthy skin, may reduce risk	Liver, eggs, whole milk, dark green leafy vegetables, yellow and orange vegetables and fruit
Vitamin B_1 (thiamin)	Water-soluble	Enzyme activity, metabolism of nutrients	Oatmeal, enriched breads and grains, rice, dairy products, fish, pork, liver, nuts, legumes
Vitamin B_2 (riboflavin)	Water-soluble	Growth, metabolism of nutrients	Dairy products, eggs, organ meats, enriched breads and grains, green leafy vegetables
Vitamin B_3 (niacin)	Water-soluble	Tissue repair, metabolism of nutrients	Organ meats, peanuts, brewer's yeast, enriched breads and grains, meats, poultry, fish and nuts
Vitamin B_6 (pyridoxine)	Water-soluble	Metabolism of nutrients (primary role)	Brewer's yeast, wheat, germ, pork, liver, whole grain cereals, potatoes, milk, fruits and vegetables
Folic Acid (part of B vitamin group)	Water-soluble	Growth, enzyme activity, prevents neural tube defects	Liver, lima and kidney beans, dark leafy vegetables, beef, potatoes, whole wheat bread
Vitamin B_{12}	Water-soluble	Metabolism of nutrients, prevents anemia	Liver, kidneys, meat, fish, dairy products, eggs
Biotin (part of B vitamin group)	Water-soluble	Enzyme activity; deficiency can lead to a type of dermatitis	Liver, milk, meat, egg yolk, vegetables, fruit, peanuts, brewer's yeast
Vitamin C	Water-soluble	Many cellular functions, promotes healthy teeth, skin and tissue repair	Citrus fruits such as oranges and grapefruits leafy vegetables, tomatoes, strawberries
Vitamin D	Fat-soluble	Essential for normal growth, development, bones and teeth	Liver, butter, fortified milk, fatty fish (fish liver oils), exposure to sunlight
Vitamin E	Fat-soluble	Antioxidant function protects cells; assists neurological function, prevents anemia	Vegetable and fish oils, nuts, seeds, egg yolk, whole grains
Vitamin K	Fat-soluble	Blood clotting	Green leafy vegetables, liver, wheat bran, tomatoes, cheese, egg yolk
Zinc	n/a	Growth and development, immune system	Meat, poultry, eggs, dairy products

Milk and dairy products provide a balance of proteins, carbohydrates and fats, and are an important source of calcium and vitamin D.

In both the US and Canada, health authorities have devised charts that recommend a range of servings from each of the four food groups. Whether it's The Food Pyramid (in the US) or Canada's Food Guide to Healthy Eating, the message is very much the same: Enjoy a variety of healthy foods every day.

Being
vegetarian

While vegetarianism has been practised in many countries for centuries, it is a relatively new (but increasingly popular) lifestyle in North America. For some people, the decision to become a vegetarian is a moral one although, for many more, the decision is motivated by health concerns. Vegetarian diets are generally perceived to be better for you – and while it's true that they can be low in saturated fat and cholesterol, this is not always the case. A vegetarian regime is typically high in dietary fiber.

It's difficult to generalize, of course, if only because "vegetarian" seems to be defined so may ways. Popular variants include *semi-vegetarians* (no red meat); *lacto-ovo vegetarians* (no meat, poultry, fish or seafood, but allows consumption of milk, milk products, and eggs); and *vegans* (no animal products of any kind – even honey in many cases).

If you are raising your child as a vegetarian, it is important to understand the nutritional implications of doing so, because these are not the same as they are for an adult. On the whole, children will grow and develop well on lacto-ovo and semi-vegetarian diets, which are sufficiently varied to meet nutrient requirements for protein, calcium, and vitamin D.

Vegan diets, however, must be carefully planned to ensure adequate intake of all essential nutrients. For example, infants on a vegan diet who are not breastfed should continue to consume fortified soy formula until they are 2 years old in order to get the additional vitamins and minerals needed – although many healthcare professionals do not recommend any kind of vegan diet for young children.

As a rule, the more restrictive a child's vegetarian diet, the more you will need to pay attention to their nutrient intake. Specific areas of concern are described below.

Protein should not be a concern for semi-vegetarians or lacto-ovo vegetarians, since their diet contains adequate amounts of animal proteins (known as complete proteins because they contain all 22 amino acids) from foods such as milk, cheese, eggs and chicken. Plant proteins, however, are incomplete proteins, which means they are deficient in one or more essential amino acids. As a result, vegans must eat a wide variety of plant proteins to make up all the amino acids they need. For example, baked beans and bread on their own do not provide one or more essential amino acids. Eaten together as part of a varied diet, however, they make up the essential amino acids the other lacks.

Vitamin B_{12} is found only in animal products, and is important for the process of cell division. A deficiency of this vitamin can lead to megaloblastic anemia, which can result in permanent neurological damage. Lacto-ovo vegetarians generally do not have difficulty consuming enough vitamin B_{12}. The equivalent of 3 cups (750 mL) milk per day or 2 cups (500 mL) milk and 1 egg per day will provide adequate vitamin B_{12} for children under the age of 2 years. Infants on a vegan diet, however, should take a vitamin B_{12} supplement of at least to 0.3 µg (micrograms) per day. The breast milk of vegan mothers can also be vitamin-B_{12} deficient, in which case both mother and infant should receive a supplement. Speak with your pediatrician or family doctor for more information.

Vitamin D is important for the development of healthy bones and teeth, and is found in fortified infant formula and cow's milk, as well as cod liver oil. All exclusively breast-fed infants, as well as children consuming a vegan diet, should receive a vitamin-D supplement to prevent deficiency. While vitamin D can be obtained through non-dietary means – that is, by exposure to sunlight – many breastfed babies in Canada and the northern U.S. do not receive enough sunlight during the day to produce adequate amounts.

Iron is essential for the formation of red blood cells. A lack of this mineral – leading to iron-deficiency anemia (see page 75) – is the most common nutritional deficiency seen in vegetarian children, especially those on a vegan diet. This is not because plant foods lack iron. In fact, dark green and orange vegetables (such as spinach and squash) are great sources of iron. The difficulty lies in the chemistry of plant-based iron, which is not as well absorbed as iron from animal-based foods. While ensuring adequate iron intake is a particular concern for vegans, it can also be important for semi- and lacto-ovo-vegetarians. For young children, this means a diet that includes iron-supplemented formula and iron-enriched infant cereal.

Calcium works with vitamin D to promote the growth of strong, healthy bones and teeth, and helps to prevent osteoporosis in later life. As such, it is important to ensure that children receive adequate dietary calcium in their growing years. Calcium intake should not be a concern for lacto-ovo- and semi-vegetarians who consume enough dairy products – typically 2 cups (500 mL) milk per day for children under 5 years. Children on a vegan diet should receive a calcium supplement in order to avoid deficiency.

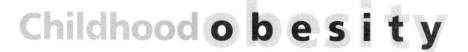

Childhood obesity

Obesity – specifically, childhood obesity – has been on the rise since 1965. In 1980, about 25% of the adult population in the US was obese, and that rate increased to 34% by 1990. It was also estimated that approximately 25% of children between the ages of 6 and 17 years were overweight or obese.

What accounts for this trend? One factor is the growing abundance and consumption of high-calorie, convenience foods. Technological growth is also partly to blame, having led to the creation of more time- and labor-saving devices, and a resulting decline in physical activity. Genetic factors also play a role in obesity, since children of obese parents are at an increased risk of becoming obese themselves.

All of these statistics may be depressingly familiar to adults – particularly those who are engaged in the difficult business of trying to lose weight. But surely, you might ask, shouldn't young children be spared such dietary restrictions?

Absolutely. While most nutritionists agree that an adult diet should consist of no more than 30% of calories from fat (and less than 10% of calories from saturated fats), these restrictions need not apply to children from birth to the age of 2 years. Indeed, during infancy a high-fat diet (about 50% of calories from fat) is actually beneficial, providing all the caloric and fatty acid intakes needed for growth and development.

The freedom from restriction can extend to the preschool years, when children have high activity levels and a fluctuating appetite. Small frequent feedings play an important role in meeting energy requirements. Preschoolers are dependent on their caregivers to make food choices for them, and healthy eating patterns and choices should be promoted – as should frequent physical exercise.

The transition from the high-fat diet of infancy to the lower-fat diet of adults should occur slowly from age 2 until adolescence, when a child has reached his or her full height. During this transition, it is important to provide children with sufficient calories to promote normal growth and development. But this also the critical period for developing healthy eating habits and a positive attitude towards food. This includes consuming a variety of foods from the four food groups, including complex carbohydrates and lower-fat foods, as well as participating in a physically active lifestyle. It is important to remember that just because an infant or toddler is chubby does not mean that he or she will grow to become an obese adult.

BETTER BABY FOOD

T I P

There is no evidence that implementing a diet of no more than 30% fat and no more than 10% saturated fat intakes will provide benefit to children and decrease the risk of heart disease later in life.

CALORIE COUNTING
Recommended energy intakes for children

Age	RDA (US)	RNI (Canada)
0 to 3 months	650 kcal/day	100 to 120 kcal/kg/day
3 to 6 months	650 kcal/day	95 to 100 kcal/kg/day
6 to 9 months	850 kcal/day	95 to 97 kcal/kg/day
9 to 12 months	850 kcal/day	97 to 99 kcal/kg/day
1 to 2 years	1300 kcal/day	101 kcal/kg/day
2 to 3 years	1300 kcal/day	94 kcal/kg/day

If you are concerned about your child's eating habits or weight or your child has a special condition (such as hyperlipidemia), speak with your doctor or a registered dietitian. Your public health department can also be a terrific source of general information on nutrition and healthy eating for infants and toddlers.

Cultural effects on diet in children

North American society has become increasingly multicultural, with the result that there is an ever wider diversity of dietary preferences and habits among families of different backgrounds. Occasionally, these can affect a young child's health. For example, in some cultures, it is not unusual to give tea to infants. But if tea is given for a prolonged period, replacing breast milk or formula, those children may become iron deficient. In other cultures, rice is a staple food for infants, which may displace iron-rich or other solid foods. Or evaporated milk may be considered a more affordable alternative to infant formula. In both cases, iron deficiency can result if supplements are not given.

Resources

- Canada's Food Guide to Healthy Eating: www.hc-sc.gc.ca/hppd/nutrition/pube/foodguid/foodguide.html

- The Food Pyramid (US): www.nal.usda.gov/fnic/Fpyr/pyramid.gif

- Melina, V; Davis, B.; and Harrison, V. *Becoming Vegetarian.* Toronto: Macmillan Canada, 1994. A good reference for vegetarian parents.

Breakfast

6 to 8 months

Makes 1 1/4 cups (300 mL)

Apple Sauce

Kitchen Tip

For infants just starting fruits, you can use a sweeter eating apple (such as Golden Delicious) and eliminate the sugar. When adding sugar, do it 1 tbsp (15 mL) at a time, tasting after each addition so applesauce does not become too sweet. For older infants, try puréeing to a thicker texture.

3	medium cooking apples, washed, peeled, cored and cut into quarters	3
2/3 cups	water	150 mL
3 tbsp	granulated sugar	45 mL

1. In a saucepan combine apples and water. Bring to a boil and cook for about 10 minutes or until apples are tender. Drain.

2. Stir in the sugar. Mash with fork to desired texture or, for a smoother texture, purée in a food processor and strain through a sieve.

NUTRITIONAL ANALYSIS per 1/4 cup (50 mL)	Energy 80 kcal	Protein 0.1 g	Carbohydrate 20.7 g	Fat 0.3 g	Iron 0.07 mg

8 to 12 months

Serves 1

Fruity Cottage Cheese

This combination makes a great breakfast or meatless lunch dish. Its very soft texture makes it ideal for children who are just starting textures.

1/4 cup	cottage cheese	50 mL
2 tbsp	chopped canned peaches	25 mL

1. In a small bowl, combine cottage cheese and peaches. Serve.

NUTRITIONAL ANALYSIS	Energy 64 kcal	Protein 6.1 g	Carbohydrate 5.1 g	Fat 2.2 g	Iron 0.16 mg

Hot Breakfast Ideas

It's nice to introduce your infant to different hot cooked cereals. It can lead to a lifetime of enjoying the pleasure and comfort of a hot cereal start to the day. These single serve amounts can be easily increased according to the child's appetite. Serve with extra milk and sugar as desired.

8 to 12 months

Each serves 1

Variations

For a treat, add a sprinkle of ground nutmeg or cinnamon. For children older than 12 months, try adding raisins and chopped dried fruit like prunes, apricots or apples are appropriate, a few to each serving during cooking.

Cooked Rolled Oats or Cream of Wheat

Microwave: In a small microwavable bowl, combine 1 tbsp (15 mL) quick cooking rolled oats with 2 tbsp (25 mL) water, milk or formula. Microwave, uncovered, on High for about 1 minute; stir. Let stand until appropriate serving temperature is reached and mixture has thickened. Stir and serve.

Stovetop: In a small saucepan, use same measurements as above. Cook, stirring frequently, over medium-low heat for 2 to 4 minutes.

NUTRITIONAL ANALYSIS	Energy	Protein	Carbohydrate	Fat	Iron
	39 kcal	1.8 g	4.9 g	1.4 g	0.23 mg

Cooked Oat Bran

Microwave: In a small microwavable bowl, combine 1 tbsp (15 mL) oat bran with 3 tbsp (45 mL) water, milk or formula. Microwave, uncovered, on High (100%) for about minute; stir. Let stand until appropriate serving temperature is reached and mixture has thickened. Stir and serve.

Stovetop: In a small saucepan, use same measurements as above. Cook, stirring frequently, over medium-low heat for 2 to 4 minutes.

NUTRITIONAL ANALYSIS	Energy	Protein	Carbohydrate	Fat	Iron
	35 kcal	2.0 g	4.0 g	1.7 g	0.47 mg

Whole Grain Cereal Mix

Combine 1/2 cup (125 mL) each: quick cooking rolled oats, oat bran and whole wheat cereal. Store in a tightly sealed container. Makes 1 1/2 cups (375 mL).

Microwave: In a small microwavable bowl, combine 1 tbsp (15 mL) cereal mix with 3 tbsp (45 mL) water, milk or formula. Microwave, uncovered, on High for about 1 minute; stir. Microwave, uncovered, on Low for 1 minute. Let stand until appropriate serving temperature is reached and mixture has thickened. Stir and serve.

Stovetop: In a small saucepan, use same measurements as above. Cook over medium-low heat for 2 to 4 minutes; stir frequently. Cover and remove from heat; let stand a few minutes.

NUTRITIONAL ANALYSIS	Energy	Protein	Carbohydrate	Fat	Iron
	48 kcal	0.4 g	6.1 g	1.8 g	0.3 mg

8 to 12 months

Serves 1

Cottage Cheese 'n' Fruit

Kitchen Tip

If you wish, substitute plain or fruit-flavored yogurt for the sour cream.

This recipe works well with many kinds of fruit. Choose the ones most popular with your infant. Serve with toast squares for a healthy breakfast.

1/4 cup	cottage cheese	50 mL
2 tbsp	sour cream (see Tip)	25 mL
1/4 cup	chopped fresh fruit (such as orange, pineapple, banana, apple, strawberry, kiwi fruit, peach, pear)	50 mL
Pinch	brown sugar	Pinch
Pinch	ground cinnamon	Pinch

1. In a small bowl, stir together cottage cheese, sour cream and fruit of your choice. Sprinkle lightly with sugar and cinnamon.

NUTRITIONAL ANALYSIS	Energy	Protein	Carbohydrate	Fat	Iron
	101 kcal	6.9 g	5.7 g	5.8 g	0.41 mg

12 to 18 months

Makes 2 cups (500 mL)

Baby's Fruit Smoothie

Kitchen Tips

Busy parents can have this smoothie ready in the refrigerator the night before to serve at breakfast. You may even find you'll enjoy it as well.

Because it contains honey, this recipe is only appropriate for children over 12 months. For younger children, replace honey with an equal quantity of granulated sugar.

Just like a milkshake – but even better.
Start with cold milk, fruit and yogurt, then blend until smooth.

1	large banana	1
1 cup	raspberries or strawberries	250 mL
3/4 cup	2% milk	175 mL
1/3 cup	plain yogurt	75 mL
1 tbsp	liquid honey (see Tip)	15 mL

1. In a blender combine banana and berries; purée until smooth. Add milk, yogurt and honey; blend for 1 minute or until smooth and frothy. Chill before serving or enjoy immediately.

NUTRITIONAL ANALYSIS	Energy	Protein	Carbohydrate	Fat	Iron
per 1/4 cup (50 mL)	44 kcal	1.4 g	8.5 g	0.9 g	0.15 mg

Fast Breakfasts

Here are a couple of fast-start recipes for those
"what am I going to feed my child for breakfast" mornings.
Each can easily be multiplied to serve the entire family.

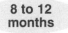

8 to 12 months

Serves 1

Fruit & Raisin Toast

1	slice raisin bread	1
1 tbsp	smooth peanut butter (see Tip)	15 mL
1/4 cup	diced apple	50 mL
Pinch	granulated sugar and ground cinnamon	Pinch

1. Toast bread, spread with peanut butter. Top with apple, fold in half so apple is secure inside. Cut into fingers and serve.

NUTRITIONAL ANALYSIS	Energy	Protein	Carbohydrate	Fat	Iron
	179 kcal	5.7 g	21.4 g	9.0 g	1.1 mg

Kitchen Tip

For a change of taste – or for children who cannot tolerate peanut butter – substitute cream cheese, a fruit spread or processed Cheddar cheese.

over 18 months

Serves 4

Pineapple Bagel
PREHEAT BROILER

1	bagel	1
2 tbsp	cream cheese	25 mL
2	slices canned pineapple, drained	2
1/2 tsp	granulated sugar	2 mL
Pinch	ground cinnamon	Pinch

1. Slice bagel in half crosswise. Spread each half with 1 tbsp (15 mL) cheese. Top each half with 1 pineapple slice; sprinkle lightly with sugar and cinnamon.

2. Place on a baking pan; broil under preheated broiler for 1 minute or until cheese starts to melt. Allow to cool slightly before cutting into child-size portions.

NUTRITIONAL ANALYSIS	Energy	Protein	Carbohydrate	Fat	Iron
per serving	123 kcal	3.5 g	21.0 g	3.0 g	0.98 mg

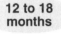

Serves 6

Makes 1 cup (250 mL)

Yogurt Orange Fruit Dip

A breakfast or healthy and tasty snack, this yogurt dip will be useful with many different fresh fruits.

Kitchen Tips

Any favorite fruit flavored yogurt may be used

Choose any fruit jam that will be compatible with the yogurt.

Food Safety Tip

When it comes to food safety, cold temperatures can keep most harmful bacteria from growing or multiplying on food.

Half	pkg (8 oz [250 g]) softened cream cheese	Half
1/2 cup	peach yogurt (see Tip)	125 mL
1/4 cup	orange marmalade (see Tip)	50 mL
1/4 tsp	vanilla or maple extract	1 mL
Pinch	ground ginger	Pinch
	Assorted fresh fruit	

1. In a small bowl, beat cream cheese, yogurt, marmalade, vanilla and ginger until blended. Spoon into a covered container and store in the refrigerator for up to 2 days.

2. Allow to soften slightly before serving with fruit.

NUTRITIONAL ANALYSIS	Energy	Protein	Carbohydrate	Fat	Iron
per 1 tbsp (15 mL)	46 kcal	0.8 g	4.5 g	2.9 g	0.12 mg

12 to 18 months

Serves 4

Orange Smoothie Shake

3/4 cup	frozen orange juice concentrate, thawed	175 mL
1 cup	2% milk	250 mL
1 cup	water	250 mL
1/4 cup	granulated sugar	50 mL
1/2 tsp	vanilla extract	2 mL
5	ice cubes	5

1. In a blender, combine orange juice concentrate, milk, water, sugar and vanilla. With motor running, add ice cubes on at a time. Blend until smooth.

NUTRITIONAL ANALYSIS	Energy	Protein	Carbohydrate	Fat	Iron
per 1 serving	156 kcal	3.4 g	33.3 g	1.4 g	0.22 mg

12 to 18
months

Serves 4

Makes 1 1/2 cups (375 mL)

Spiced Banana Sauce

This topping is excellent for pancakes, frozen waffles or French toast. It combines two all-time child favorites – bananas and cream cheese.

Variations

Pineapple Sauce: Replace banana with 1/2 cup (125 mL) drained canned crushed pineapple.

Strawberry Sauce: Replace banana with 1 1/2 cups (375 mL) sliced strawberries.

Serving Suggestion

Cut pancakes, waffles or French toast into baby-bite-size pieces. Top with sauce.

2 tbsp	frozen orange juice concentrate, thawed	25 mL
2 tbsp	water	25 mL
1/4 cup	cream cheese (at room temperature)	50 mL
1/2 to 1 tsp	granulated sugar	2 to 5 mL
1/8 tsp	ground cinnamon	0.5 mL
1/8 tsp	ground nutmeg	0.5 mL
2	bananas, cut into slices	2
	Frozen waffles	

1. In a small nonstick skillet, combine orange juice, water, cream cheese, sugar, cinnamon and nutmeg. Cook over medium heat for about 5 minutes or until heated and smooth; stir frequently. Add bananas and cook for 1 minute until slices are coated with sauce.

2. Toast waffles. Spoon some warm sauce over each.

NUTRITIONAL ANALYSIS	Energy	Protein	Carbohydrate	Fat	Iron
per 1/4 cup (50 mL)	74 kcal	1.1 g	11.7 g	3.1 g	0.3 mg

12 to 18 months

Serves 6
Makes 1 cup (250 mL)

Ricotta Cream Sauce

Enjoy this sauce as a breakfast fruit dip or serve over cut-up fresh fruit at another meal.

1 cup	smooth 2% ricotta cheese	250 mL
2 tbsp	confectioner's (icing) sugar	25 mL
1 tsp	grated orange zest	5 mL
1/2 tsp	vanilla extract	2 mL

Fresh fruit pieces (banana chunks,
seedless grapes, melon pieces,
whole strawberries,
kiwi slices, or any other fresh
fruit suitable for dipping)

1. In a small bowl, beat together cheese and sugar until smooth. Stir in orange zest and vanilla. Spoon into a tightly sealed container and store in the refrigerator for up to 1 week.

2. Serve in a small container suitable for dipping fruit.

NUTRITIONAL ANALYSIS	Energy	Protein	Carbohydrate	Fat	Iron
per 1 tbsp (15 mL)	25 kcal	1.8 g	1.6 g	1.2 g	0.07 mg

Basic Fast Fruit Sauce

Serves 6

Makes 2 1/3 cups (575 mL)

Kitchen Tip

Prepared fruits are stemmed, pitted, peeled (if necessary) and sliced.

Food Safety Tip

All produce should be washed under cool running water prior to eating or cooking.

Both children and adults will love these fruit sauces. They make handy toppings for pancakes, milk or rice pudding, cottage cheese or ice cream or other fresh fruits. Use your favorite fruits when they are at their freshest best. Make lots of sauce and freeze what you can't use now.

2 cups	prepared fruit, such as strawberries, blueberries, raspberries, Saskatoon berries, pitted sour cherries, peaches and plums (see Tip)	500 mL
1 cup	water, divided	250 mL
2 tbsp	cornstarch	25 mL
1/2 cup	granulated sugar (or more to taste)	125 mL
1 tbsp	lemon juice	15 mL

1. In a saucepan, bring 3/4 cup (175 mL) of the water to a boil. Add fruit. Return to a boil, reduce heat to low and cook, uncovered, for 5 minutes.

2. Blend together cornstarch, sugar and remaining 1/4 cup (50 mL) water. Add slowly to fruit and boil until thick and clear, stirring constantly. Taste for sweetness – extra sugar may be added now.

3. Stir lemon juice into fruit. Sauce may be served warm or cooled and stored in the refrigerator.

NUTRITIONAL ANALYSIS	Energy	Protein	Carbohydrate	Fat	Iron
per 1 tbsp (15 mL)	14 kcal	0.1 g	3.7 g	0.0 g	0.03 mg

12 to 18 months

Serves 2

Iron-Boosted Oatmeal

This oatmeal is not only a great source of iron, but its thick, "stay in the spoon" consistency makes it easy for children to feed themselves.

2/3 cup	water	150 mL
1/3 cup	oatmeal (quick-cooking variety)	75 mL
1/8 tsp	salt	0.5 mL
3 tbsp	infant rice cereal (iron-fortified)	45 mL
2 tbsp	whole milk	25 mL
2 tsp	brown sugar	10 mL

1. In a large saucepan, bring water to a boil. Add oatmeal and salt; return to a boil, reduce heat and simmer for 3 to 5 minutes. Stir in rice cereal and milk (adjust quantities, if you wish, to achieve desired consistency). Sprinkle with brown sugar. Allow to cool before serving.

NUTRITIONAL ANALYSIS	Energy	Protein	Carbohydrate	Fat	Iron
per serving	89 kcal	2.9 g	16.2 g	1.5 g	2.34 mg

12 to 18 months

Makes 16

Oatmeal Pancakes

These whole grain pancakes will be enjoyed by young and the not-so-young alike. Try them plain, with syrup, or with a topping of fresh fruit with fruit-flavored yogurt.

Kitchen Tips

To avoid tough-textured pancakes, be sure you don't overmix the batter. Allow the batter to sit for a few minutes before cooking.

Cook all pancake batter, then freeze pancakes by separating each between sheets of waxed paper. These will make a fast-start meal another day.

1 1/4 cups	whole wheat flour	300 mL
3/4 cup	rolled oats	175 mL
1/4 cup	wheat germ	50 mL
1/4 cup	instant skim milk powder	50 mL
2 tbsp	packed brown sugar	25 mL
1 tsp	baking powder	5 mL
1/4 tsp	salt	1 mL
2	eggs, lightly beaten	2
2 cups	buttermilk	500 mL
1/4 cup	vegetable oil, divided	50 mL

1. In a medium bowl, combine flour, rolled oats, wheat germ, milk powder, sugar, baking powder and salt.

2. In a second bowl, beat together eggs, buttermilk and 3 tbsp (45 mL) of the oil. Pour into dry ingredients; stir just until moistened.

3. In a nonstick skillet over medium heat, warm 1 tbsp (15 mL) oil until hot. Using a 1/4-cup (50 mL) measure, pour batter into hot skillet; cook for 3 minutes or until bubbles break on surface and underside is golden brown. Turn pancakes with a spatula and cook just until bottom is lightly browned. Repeat with remaining batter.

NUTRITIONAL ANALYSIS	Energy	Protein	Carbohydrate	Fat	Iron
per pancake	110 kcal	4.7 g	13.6 g	4.5 g	0.8 mg

Egg Starters

The following quick egg ideas make ideal breakfasts or lunches for your child. Add a light sprinkle of chopped parsley for visual appeal. Enjoy the same meal with your child by doubling any of the recipes for an adult helping.

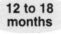

12 to 18 months

Serves 1

Egg and Cottage Cheese

1 tsp	butter *or* margarine	5 mL
1	egg	1
1 tbsp	cottage cheese	15 mL

Salt and freshly ground black pepper to taste

1. In a small skillet, melt butter over medium-low heat.
2. In a small bowl, stir together egg and cottage cheese. Pour into skillet; cook, stirring frequently, until egg is cooked to desired consistency. Lightly season to taste with salt and pepper.

Variations

Replace cottage cheese with 1 tbsp (15 mL) grated Cheddar, mozzarella, Swiss, Monterey Jack, ricotta, diced tofu or other available cheese.

NUTRITIONAL ANALYSIS	Energy	Protein	Carbohydrate	Fat	Iron
	129 kcal	7.9 g	1.3 g	10.1 g	1.2 mg

12 to 18 months

Serves 1

Scrambled Egg with Asparagus

1 tsp	butter *or* margarine	5 mL
1 tsp	finely chopped onion	5 mL
1	egg, lightly beaten	1
1 tbsp	whole milk	15 mL
1	stalk cooked asparagus, cut into small pieces	1

1. In a small skillet, melt butter over medium-low heat. Add onion and sauté for 1 minute or until softened.
2. Whisk egg with milk; add to skillet. Cook, stirring frequently, until egg is cooked to desired consistency. Top with asparagus pieces, cover and remove from heat. Allow to stand a few minutes until asparagus is warm. Lightly season to taste with salt and pepper.

Vegetable Variations

Replace asparagus with other cooked vegetables, such as small amounts of chopped carrot, green beans, broccoli, corn kernels, red or green bell pepper, chopped tomato or mashed sweet potatoes.

NUTRITIONAL ANALYSIS	Energy	Protein	Carbohydrate	Fat	Iron
	127 kcal	7.1 g	2.5 g	9.8 g	1.3 mg

Serves 1

Egg in a Hole

Kitchen Tip

Some children may prefer this dish without cheese. Try it both ways.

Here we have egg and toast in one convenient package that tastes great. It's an old favorite that never goes out of style.

1	slice whole wheat bread	1
1 tsp	butter *or* margarine	5 mL
1	medium egg	1
1 tbsp	shredded Cheddar cheese (see Tip)	15 mL

1. Using a cookie cutter or the rim of a glass, cut a circle from middle of bread.

2. In nonstick skillet, melt butter over medium-low heat. Place bread and bread round separately in skillet. Break egg into hole, cover skillet and cook for 5 minutes or until egg is almost set. Sprinkle with cheese. Continue to cook until cheese starts to melt. Top with bread round and serve.

NUTRITIONAL ANALYSIS	Energy	Protein	Carbohydrate	Fat	Iron
per serving	195 kcal	9.2 g	14.7 g	11.5 g	1.78 mg

12 to 18 months

Serves 4

Makes 8 slices

Overnight French Toast

Children love toast – so they'll really enjoy this "toast with an egg twist." (Parents will enjoy this classic breakfast dish too!) French toast is normally quite time consuming, and is hard to fit into busy morning schedules. So try this overnight version. Accompany it with a fruit sauce or maple syrup, or just serve it plain and enjoy its marvelous flavor and crisp texture alone.

2	eggs	2
1 tbsp	granulated sugar	15 mL
1/2 cup	whole milk	125 mL
1/2 tsp	grated orange zest	2 mL
1/4 tsp	ground cinnamon	1 mL
8	slices French bread stick	8
1 tbsp	butter *or* margarine	15 mL

1. In a small bowl, whisk together eggs, sugar, milk, orange rind and cinnamon until blended.

2. Place bread slices in a shallow baking dish large enough to hold the 8 slices in a single layer. Pour egg mixture evenly over bread, turn each slice to coat. Cover and refrigerate overnight.

3. Heat butter in a large nonstick skillet over medium-high heat. Add bread; cook for 2 minutes per side or until each side is golden brown.

NUTRITIONAL ANALYSIS	Energy	Protein	Carbohydrate	Fat	Iron
per slice	130 kcal	4.8 g	19.5 g	3.4 g	1.05 mg

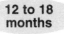

12 to 18 months

Serves 4

Mushroom Scrambled Eggs

Food Safety Tip

Bacteria are found on all raw agricultural products. Wash all produce under cool running water prior to eating or cooking.

Enjoy this flavorful egg recipe on mornings when you have a little more time to cook. It is easy to serve just the right amount for infant appetites.

4	eggs, beaten	4
3 tbsp	whole milk	45 mL
1/4 tsp	salt	1 mL
Pinch	freshly ground black pepper	Pinch
1 tbsp	butter *or* margarine	15 mL
1	green onion, thinly sliced	1
1 cup	sliced mushrooms	250 mL

1. In a small bowl, whisk together eggs, milk, salt and pepper; set aside.

2. In a large nonstick skillet, melt butter over medium-high heat. Add onions and mushrooms; cook, stirring frequently, for 2 minutes or until just tender.

3. Reduce heat to medium-low. Pour egg mixture into skillet. Cook for 3 minutes, stirring frequently, or until eggs begin to set. Continue to cook until eggs reach desired consistency.

NUTRITIONAL ANALYSIS	Energy	Protein	Carbohydrate	Fat	Iron
per serving	115 kcal	6.9 g	2.1 g	8.8 g	1.35 mg

12 to 18 months

Serves 1 or 2

Quick Cheese Omelet

Serve this fast and easy dish with toast, a bagel or an English muffin.

1	egg	1
1 tbsp	whole milk	15 mL
1 oz	Cheddar cheese, cut into 1-inch (2.5 cm) pieces	25 g

1. In a small microwave-safe dish, whisk together egg and milk. Add cheese.

2. Microwave, uncovered, on High for 1 1/2 to 2 minutes, stirring at the halfway point to ensure that all of egg is cooked. (Actual cooking time will vary according to the power of your microwave.) Let stand for 5 minutes before serving.

NUTRITIONAL ANALYSIS	Energy	Protein	Carbohydrate	Fat	Iron
per recipe	209 kcal	14.1 g	1.7 g	16.0 g	1.29 mg

12 to 18 months

Serves 4 Adults
Makes 12 Baby Servings

Overnight Cheese Strata

Kitchen Tip

Add your choice of assorted chopped vegetables – such as sliced mushrooms, broccoli florets, red or green bell peppers. Arrange over bread cubes in Step 1 and proceed with recipe.

Food Safety Tip

Refrigerate leftovers within 2 hours. This is one simple way that you can give bacteria the cold shoulder!

Make this terrific recipe the night before, then pop into the oven about 30 minutes before serving. Useful when weekend guests are expected. Allow small cubes of the strata to cool before serving to little fingers and mouths.

PREHEAT OVEN TO 350° F (180° C)
13- BY 9-INCH (3.5 L) BAKING PAN, GREASED

6	slices whole wheat or white bread, crusts removed	6
2 cups	shredded medium Cheddar cheese, divided	500 mL
6	eggs, beaten	6
2 cups	2% milk	500 mL
2	green onions, sliced	2
1/2 tsp	dried oregano	2 mL
1/2 tsp	salt	2 mL
1/4 tsp	freshly ground black pepper	1 mL
1	large tomato, cut into wedges	1
	Chopped fresh parsley	

1. Cut bread into cubes. Arrange cubes in prepared baking dish. Sprinkle with one-half the cheese.

2. In a medium bowl, combine eggs, milk, onions, oregano, salt and pepper. Pour over bread. Sprinkle with remaining cheese. Cover with plastic wrap and refrigerate for several hours or overnight.

3. Arrange tomato wedges on top of strata. Bake in preheated oven for 35 minutes or until light golden brown and center is set. Let stand for 5 minutes before cutting into squares.

NUTRITIONAL ANALYSIS	Energy	Protein	Carbohydrate	Fat	Iron
per baby serving	274 kcal	16.8 g	10.5 g	18.5 g	1.38 mg

12 to 18 months

Serves 4

Microwave Breakfast Eggs Florentine

Kitchen Tip

If there are only 3 people in the family, you may want to reserve some of the spinach mixture for another meal.

This recipe may be too much to prepare during the week, but a lazy weekend would be the perfect time to enjoy it. And it's a great way to start the wee ones appreciating fine dining.

1	pkg (10 oz [300 g]) frozen chopped spinach, thawed	1
2 tbsp	finely chopped onion	25 mL
4	eggs	4
1 tbsp	grated Parmesan cheese	15 mL
1/4 tsp	salt	1 mL
1/4 tsp	dried basil	1 mL
4	English muffins, halved	4

1. Squeeze excess moisture from spinach.

2. In a small microwavable bowl, combine spinach and onion. Cover and microwave on High for 3 minutes. Spoon mixture into 4 medium-size custard cups, using more spinach for adult servings (see Tip).

3. Break 1 egg into each dish; pierce with a fork. Sprinkle with cheese, salt and basil. Cover and microwave on Medium-High for 6 minutes or until eggs are cooked to desired consistency.

4. Meanwhile, toast muffin halves. Using a rubber spatula, slide cooked egg and spinach onto muffin halves. Serve with second muffin half.

NUTRITIONAL ANALYSIS	Energy	Protein	Carbohydrate	Fat	Iron
per serving	249 kcal	13.6 g	32.1 g	7.4 g	4.40 mg

Serves 1

Ham and Egg Muffin

PREHEAT OVEN TO 350° F (180° C)
MUFFIN TIN

Kitchen Tip

To prevent the muffin tin from warping, place a little water in each unused cup before placing in oven.

1	slice bread	1
1 tsp	butter *or* margarine	5 mL
1	slice ham, chopped	1
1	egg	1
1 tbsp	grated Cheddar cheese	15 mL

1. Remove crusts from bread and butter one side. Press bread into muffin tin, butter-side down. Insert ham pieces and egg. Top with cheese. Bake 15 minutes until egg is cooked.

NUTRITIONAL ANALYSIS	Energy	Protein	Carbohydrate	Fat	Iron
per muffin	307 kcal	17.7 g	15.8 g	18.7 g	2.19 mg

Makes 12

BREAKFAST

Apple Breakfast Bars

These moist, fruit-filled bars make a nice change from muffins.

Kitchen Tip

If you can't find date snacking cake, use another variety. Make sure the package size is the same and that it does not contain nuts.

PREHEAT OVEN TO 350° F (180° C)

9-INCH (2 L) SQUARE CAKE PAN, GREASED

3 cups	finely chopped, peeled apples, divided (about 2 large apples)	750 mL
1	pkg (14 oz [400 g]) date snacking cake mix (see Tip)	1
1/4 cup	wheat germ	50 mL
1/4 cup	natural wheat bran	50 mL
1 tsp	ground cinnamon	5 mL
1 cup	2% milk	250 mL
2 tbsp	brown sugar	25 mL

1. In a medium bowl, stir together 2 cups (500 mL) apples, cake mix, wheat germ, bran and cinnamon; stir in milk just until blended. Spread into cake pan.

2. Top with remaining apples; sprinkle with sugar.

3. Bake in preheated oven for 45 minutes or until tester inserted in center comes out clean. Move to wire rack to cool. Cut into bars.

NUTRITIONAL ANALYSIS	Energy	Protein	Carbohydrate	Fat	Iron
per bar	201 kcal	2.7 g	36.9 g	5.4 g	1.20 mg

Oat Bran Applesauce Muffins

Nourishing oat bran in combination with applesauce makes a healthy breakfast wake-up for all ages. If you or your little one are feeling a bit peckish between meals, these muffins are also an ideal snack with milk or juice.

PREHEAT OVEN TO 350° F (180° C)
12-CUP MUFFIN TIN, GREASED OR PAPER-LINED

1 1/3 cups	whole wheat flour	325 mL
1/2 cup	oat bran	125 mL
1/2 cup	loosely packed brown sugar	125 mL
2 tsp	baking powder	10 mL
1/2 tsp	baking soda	2 mL
1/2 tsp	ground cinnamon	2 mL
1/2 tsp	ground nutmeg	2 mL
1/4 cup	vegetable oil	50 mL
1 cup	applesauce	250 mL
1	egg, beaten	1
1/4 cup	finely chopped raisins (optional)	50 mL

1. In a large bowl, combine flour, oat bran, brown sugar, baking powder, baking soda and spices.

2. In another bowl, stir together oil, applesauce and egg. Stir in raisins. Add applesauce mixture to dry ingredients; stir just until moistened.

3. Spoon batter into prepared muffin cups. Bake in pre-heated oven for 15 minutes, or until muffins are firm to the touch. Cool 10 minutes before removing from pan to wire rack to cool completely.

NUTRITIONAL ANALYSIS	Energy	Protein	Carbohydrate	Fat	Iron
per muffin	133 kcal	2.8 g	22.0 g	4.7 g	1.19 mg

12 to 18 months

Makes 12

Banana Oat Muffins

Kitchen Tips

Because it contains honey, this recipe is only appropriate for children over 12 months. For younger children, replace honey with an equal quantity of granulated sugar.

Honey does not stick to the measuring cup if oil is measured first.

Don't have buttermilk? Sour milk makes a good substitute and it's easy to make: For the quantity needed in this recipe, add 1 1/2 tsp (7 mL) lemon juice or vinegar to a measuring cup, then add enough milk to make up 3/4 cup (175 mL); let mixture stand for 5 minutes.

Most people enjoy muffins for breakfast or as a snack – and kids are no exception. Rolled oats add extra fiber to these tasty-healthy muffins.

PREHEAT OVEN TO 400° F (200° C)

12-CUP MUFFIN TIN, GREASED OR PAPER-LINED

1 cup	all-purpose flour	250 mL
1/2 cup	whole wheat flour	125 mL
1/2 cup	rolled oats	125 mL
1 tsp	baking powder	5 mL
1/2 tsp	baking soda	2 mL
1/2 tsp	ground cinnamon	2 mL
3/4 cup	buttermilk *or* sour milk (see Tip)	175 mL
1/4 cup	vegetable oil	50 mL
1	egg	1
1/3 cup	liquid honey (see Tip)	75 mL
1	medium banana, mashed	1

1. In a large bowl, combine all-purpose and whole wheat flour, rolled oats, baking powder, baking soda and cinnamon.

2. In another bowl, combine buttermilk, oil, egg, honey and banana. Add to dry ingredients; stir just until moistened.

3. Spoon batter into prepared muffin cups. Bake in preheated oven for 18 minutes, or until muffins are firm to the touch.

NUTRITIONAL ANALYSIS	Energy	Protein	Carbohydrate	Fat	Iron
per muffin	172 kcal	4.2 g	28.7 g	5.1 g	1.49 mg

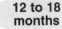

**12 to 18
months**

Makes one 12-slice loaf

Honey Loaf

Kitchen Tip

Because it contains honey, this recipe is only appropriate for children over 12 months. For younger children, use maple syrup instead of the honey.

PREHEAT OVEN TO 350° F (180° C)
9- BY 5-INCH (2 L) LOAF PAN, LIGHTLY GREASED

1/2 cup	butter *or* margarine	125 mL
1/2 cup	granulated sugar	125 mL
1	egg	1
1/3 cup	liquid honey	75 mL
1 tsp	salt	5 mL
2 1/2 cups	all-purpose flour	625 mL
1 tbsp	baking powder	15 mL
2/3 cup	2% milk	150 mL

1. In a large bowl, cream together butter and sugar. Add egg, honey and salt; mix well.

2. In another smaller bowl, combine flour and baking powder; add to butter mixture. Add milk, stirring, until just moistened.

3. Pour into prepared loaf pan and bake in preheated oven for 1 1/4 hours.

NUTRITIONAL ANALYSIS	Energy	Protein	Carbohydrate	Fat	Iron
per slice	252 kcal	3.9 g	39.2 g	9.1 g	1.23 mg

over 18 months

Makes 36

Bran Muffins

PREHEAT OVEN TO 375° F (190° C)

12-CUP MUFFIN TINS, GREASED OR PAPER-LINED

Kitchen Tip

For the quantity of sour milk needed in this recipe, add 4 tsp (20 mL) lemon juice or vinegar to a 2-cup (500 mL) measuring cup, then fill with milk; let mixture stand for 5 minutes.

2 3/4 cups	all-purpose flour	775 mL
1 1/2 cups	natural bran	375 mL
2 tsp	baking powder	10 mL
2 tsp	baking soda	10 mL
1/2 tsp	salt	2 mL
1 cup	soft margarine	250 mL
1 cup	lightly packed brown sugar	250 mL
2 cups	sour milk	500 mL
1/2 cup	raisins	125 mL
1/4 cup	molasses	50 mL
2	eggs (well beaten)	2

1. In a large bowl, combine flour, bran, baking powder, baking soda and salt.

2. In another bowl, cream together margarine and brown sugar. Add sour milk, raisins and molasses; stir until just combined. Fold in beaten eggs. Add to dry ingredients; stir just until moistened.

3. Spoon batter into prepared muffin tins. Bake in preheated oven for about 20 minutes or until browned. Allow to cool for 5 minutes before removing muffins from tins.

NUTRITIONAL ANALYSIS	Energy	Protein	Carbohydrate	Fat	Iron
per muffin	133 kcal	2.5 g	17.8 g	6.2 g	1.38 mg

Lunch

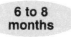

6 to 8 months

Serves 1 or 2

Puréed Baby Fruit

Kitchen Tip

Vegetable and fruit purées will keep in the freezer for 4 to 6 months. Be sure to label with date before freezing.

1/3 to 1/2 cup	cooked fruit, chopped into small pieces	75 to 125 mL
2 tsp	water or fruit juice	10 mL

1. In a small bowl, microwave fruit on High for about 1 minute. Stir in water. Transfer to a food processor or blender; process for 30 to 60 seconds until purée is smooth.

2. Serve immediately or freeze in an ice cube tray for future use.

NUTRITIONAL ANALYSIS - varies with fruit used.

6 to 8 months

Serves 3 or 4

Puréed Baby Vegetables

3/4 cup	cooked vegetables, chopped into small pieces	175 mL
3 tbsp	water or cooking liquid	45 mL

1. In a small bowl, microwave vegetables on High for about 1 minute or until tender. Stir in water. Transfer to a food processor or blender; process for 1 to 2 minutes until purée is smooth.

2. Serve immediately or freeze in an ice cube tray for future use.

NUTRITIONAL ANALYSIS - varies with vegetables used.

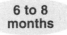

6 to 8 months

Makes 1/2 cup (125 mL)

Puréed Peaches

2	small peaches, peeled, pitted and cut into small pieces (about 1 cup [250 mL])	2
1 to 2 tsp	water	5 to 10 mL

1. In a saucepan of boiling water, cook peaches for about 10 minutes or until tender. Drain. Transfer to a food processor or blender; process for 30 to 60 seconds, adding water as needed until purée is smooth.

2. Serve immediately or freeze in an ice cube tray for future use.

6 to 8 months

Makes 1/2 cup (125 mL)

Puréed Pears

Kitchen Tip

This recipe makes enough for about half an ice cube tray. Try different varieties of pears for different flavors.

1	medium pear, peeled, cored and cut into small pieces (about 1 cup [250 mL])	1
1 to 2 tsp	water	5 to 10 mL

1. In a saucepan of boiling water, cook pear for about 15 minutes or until tender. Drain. Transfer to a food processor or blender; process for 30 to 60 seconds, adding water as needed until purée is smooth.

2. Serve immediately or freeze in an ice cube tray for future use.

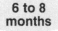

6 to 8 months

Makes 1/2 cup (125 mL)

Puréed Green Beans

Kitchen Tip

This recipe makes enough for about half an ice cube tray. Frozen or fresh varieties of beans work equally well.

1 cup	chopped green beans (washed and trimmed)	250 mL
2 tbsp	water	25 mL

1. In a saucepan of boiling water, cook beans for about 15 minutes or until tender. Drain. Transfer to a food processor or blender; process for 30 to 60 seconds, adding water as needed until purée is smooth.

2. Serve immediately or freeze in an ice cube tray for future use.

6 to 8 months

Makes 1/2 cup (125 mL)

Puréed Carrots

2	medium carrots, peeled and thinly sliced (about 1 cup [250 mL])	2
2 tbsp	water	25 mL

1. In a saucepan of boiling water, cook carrots for 12 to 15 minutes or until tender. Drain. Transfer to a food processor or blender; process for 30 to 60 seconds, adding water as needed until purée is smooth.

2. Serve immediately or freeze in an ice cube tray for future use.

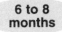

**6 to 8
months**

Makes 1/2 cup (125 mL)

Puréed Broccoli

Kitchen Tips

This recipe makes enough for about half an ice cube tray.

Try steaming broccoli instead of boiling it – more vitamins will be retained as a result.

1 cup	chopped broccoli florets (washed and trimmed)	250 mL
2 tbsp	water	25 mL

1. In a saucepan of boiling water, cook broccoli for 5 to 10 minutes or until tender. Drain. Transfer to a food processor or blender; process for 30 to 60 seconds, adding water as needed until purée is smooth.

2. Serve immediately or freeze in an ice cube tray for future use.

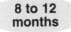

**8 to 12
months**

Makes 8 cups (2 L)

Chicken Stock

Kitchen Tip

You can purchase stewing chickens specifically for the purpose of making stock or you can also use a leftover carcass from a chicken or turkey dinner.

It is always nice to have homemade chicken, or beef stocks on hand for soups or other recipes. It freezes well and will defrost overnight.

12-CUP (3 L) STOCKPOT

2 lbs	chicken pieces and/or bones	1 kg
1	onion, thinly sliced	1
1	stalk celery, sliced	1
8 cups	cold water	2 L
	Salt and freshly ground black pepper to taste	
1	sprig parsley	1

1. Add all ingredients to stockpot and bring to a boil. Reduce heat, cover and simmer for 2 1/2 to 3 hours. Drain through a sieve to remove solids.

8 to 12 months

LUNCH

Makes 3 1/2 cups (875 mL)

Barley Vegetable Soup

As it cooks, the soup mix thickens the liquid making this hearty soup more like a stew. Prepare during morning naptime to have ready for lunch. For infants, purée until smooth. Toddlers and their elders will love it straight from the pot.

Kitchen Tip

Purchase pre-mixed bags of assorted dried legumes or mix your own.

Food Safety Tip

Bacteria thrive in foods left out at room temperature. To reduce the chance of food-borne illnesses, refrigerate any leftover soup within 2 hours.

3 cups	water	750 mL
1/3 cup	mixed dried lentils, split peas, barley (see Tip)	75 mL
1	bouillon cube, beef or vegetable	1
1	medium carrot, diced	1
1	medium potato, diced	1
1	stalk celery, chopped	1
1/2 cup	tomato sauce	125 mL
1/2 tsp	dried basil	2 mL

1. In a large saucepan, combine water, soup mix, bouillon cube, carrot, potato and celery. Bring to a boil, reduce heat and simmer, covered, for about 1 hour or until legumes are tender. Add more water if soup is too thick.

2. Add tomato sauce and basil. Heat until warmed through.

NUTRITIONAL ANALYSIS	Energy	Protein	Carbohydrate	Fat	Iron
per 1/2 cup (125 mL)	34 kcal	1.2 g	7.6 g	0.2 g	0.36 mg

12 to 18 months

Makes 4 3/4 cups (1.2 L)

Broccoli Soup

Kitchen Tip

This recipe can be prepared in advance, up to the point of adding milk in Step 3. Purée can be frozen in portion sizes until ready to eat. Just defrost and add milk; season to taste with salt and pepper. Warm until heated through.

1 tbsp	butter *or* margarine	15 mL
Half	onion, chopped	Half
1 lb	broccoli, chopped	500 g
2 cups	chicken stock, divided	500 mL
2 tbsp	all-purpose flour	25 mL
1 cup	water	250 mL
1	bay leaf	1
2 tbsp	chopped parsley	25 mL
1 cup	whole milk	250 mL
1/4 tsp	salt	1 mL
1/4 tsp	freshly ground black pepper	1 mL

1. In a large saucepan, melt butter over medium heat. Add onion and cook for about 5 minutes or until soft. Add broccoli and a few tablespoons of the chicken stock; cook, covered, for another 10 minutes. Sprinkle flour over mixture and blend well.

2. In a medium bowl, combine remaining chicken stock with water. Stir mixture into saucepan with bay leaf and parsley; cook, covered, for about 20 minutes longer. Remove and discard bay leaf.

3. Transfer soup to a food processor or blender; purée until smooth. Return mixture to saucepan and stir in milk, salt and pepper. Cook over medium-low heat for about 5 minutes or until heated through.

NUTRITIONAL ANALYSIS	Energy	Protein	Carbohydrate	Fat	Iron
per 1/2 cup (125 mL)	58 kcal	3.8 g	5.7 g	2.7 g	0.74 mg

12 to 18 months

Makes 8 cups (2 L)

Colorful Carrot Soup

Kitchen Tips

For additional protein, add tofu or cheese to soup. Serve with hot bread or buns.

This recipe can be prepared in advance, up to the point of adding milk in Step 2. Purée can be frozen in portion sizes until ready to eat. Just defrost and add milk. Warm until heated through.

For a richer texture, use cream instead of milk.

2 tbsp	butter *or* margarine	25 mL
1 cup	finely chopped onions	250 mL
3 cups	thickly sliced carrots	750 mL
4 cups	chicken stock	1 L
2 tbsp	tomato paste	25 mL
2 tbsp	long grain rice	25 mL
1/2 cup	whole milk	125 mL
1/4 tsp	salt	1 mL
1/4 tsp	freshly ground black pepper	1 mL
2 cups	water	500 mL

1. In a large skillet, melt butter over medium heat. Add onions and cook until soft. Add carrots, stock, paste and rice; reduce heat and simmer for 30 minutes.

2. In a food processor or blender, purée soup in batches until smooth, transferring each batch to a saucepan. Stir in milk, salt and pepper. Add water. Heat until warmed through before serving.

NUTRITIONAL ANALYSIS	Energy	Protein	Carbohydrate	Fat	Iron
per 1/2 cup (125 mL)	46 kcal	2.0 g	4.8 g	2.2 g	0.32 mg

Serves 4
Makes 3 cups (750 mL)

Corn Chowder

Great corn chowder was never easier than this!

1	can (10 oz [284 mL]) cream of potato soup	1
1/2 cup	2% milk	125 mL
1/2 cup	canned cream-style corn	125 mL
1	small seeded and diced tomato	1
1/4 tsp	dried thyme	1 mL
1/8 tsp	freshly ground black pepper	0.5 mL
1/4 cup	shredded Cheddar or Monterey Jack cheese	50 mL

1. In a medium saucepan, combine soup, milk, corn, tomato, thyme and pepper. Bring to a boil, stirring constantly. Spoon into serving bowls. Sprinkle each with 1 tbsp (15 mL) cheese. Allow infant servings to cool to a safe temperature.

NUTRITIONAL ANALYSIS	Energy	Protein	Carbohydrate	Fat	Iron
per 1/2 cup (125 mL)	95 kcal	4.1 g	10.6 g	4.4 g	0.51 mg

Spinach Soup

Makes 3 1/3 cups (825 mL)

Kitchen Tip

This recipe can be prepared in advance, up to the point of adding milk in Step 2. Purée can be frozen in portion sizes until ready to eat. Just defrost and add milk; season to taste with salt and pepper. Warm until heated through.

1 tbsp	butter *or* margarine	15 mL
Half	medium onion, chopped	Half
1	pkg (10 oz [284 mL] fresh spinach, washed, coarse stems removed	1
2 tbsp	all-purpose flour	25 mL
2 cups	chicken stock	500 mL
1	bay leaf	1
2 tbsp	chopped parsley	25 mL
1 cup	whole milk	250 mL
	Salt and freshly ground black pepper to taste	

1. In a large saucepan, melt butter over medium heat. Add onion and cook for about 5 minutes or until soft. Add spinach and cook, covered, for about 10 minutes longer. Sprinkle flour over mixture. Blend well. Add chicken stock, bay leaf and parsley; cook, uncovered, for about 15 minutes longer. Remove and discard bay leaf.

2. In a food processor or blender, purée soup in batches until smooth, transferring each batch to a saucepan. Stir in milk, salt and pepper. Heat until warmed through before serving.

NUTRITIONAL ANALYSIS	Energy	Protein	Carbohydrate	Fat	Iron
per 1/2 cup (125 mL)	68 kcal	4.1 g	5.7 g	3.4 g	1.46 mg

12 to 18 months

Makes 4 cups (1 L)

Vegetable Lentil Soup

Kitchen Tips

Chicken stock can be replaced by an equal quantity of canned chicken broth, or water mixed with chicken bouillon cubes or sachets. In the latter case, extra salt may not be needed.

For faster cooking time, use red lentils rather than brown or green ones.

Serving Suggestion

For extra calcium (and flavor) add a spoonful of plain yogurt or sour cream to each bowl.

Younger children may prefer this soup puréed in a blender or food processor for a smoother consistency.

1 cup	shredded carrots	250 mL
Half	small onion, finely chopped	Half
1 cup	diced rutabaga or turnip	250 mL
1	small potato, cubed	1
1	clove garlic, minced	1
1/2 cup	red lentils (see Tip)	125 mL
3 cups	chicken stock (see Tip)	750 mL
1	bay leaf	1
	Salt and freshly ground black pepper	

1. In a large saucepan, combine carrots, onion, rutabaga, potato, garlic, lentils, broth and bay leaf. Bring to a boil. Reduce heat to low and simmer, covered, for 20 minutes or until vegetables and lentils are tender. Season to taste with salt and pepper. Remove and discard bay leaf before serving.

NUTRITIONAL ANALYSIS	Energy	Protein	Carbohydrate	Fat	Iron
per 1/2 cup (125 mL)	87 kcal	6.2 g	14.2 g	0.8 g	1.60 mg

Makes 5 1/2 cups (1.375 L)
Serves 5

Fantastic Black Bean Soup

Kitchen Tip

For a refreshing flavor, try adding plain yogurt or sour cream just before serving.

2 tsp	vegetable oil	10 mL
2 tsp	minced garlic	10 mL
1 cup	chopped onions	250 mL
1 cup	chopped carrots	250 mL
1	can (19 oz [540 mL]) black beans rinsed and drained	1
3 cups	chicken stock	750 mL
3/4 tsp	ground cumin	4 mL
1/4 cup	chopped parsley	50 mL

1. In a large skillet, heat oil over medium-high heat. Add garlic, onions and carrots; cook for 4 to 5 minutes or until onions are softened. Stir in beans, chicken stock and cumin; bring to a boil. Reduce heat to medium-low and simmer, covered, for about 20 to 25 minutes or until the carrots are soft.

2. In a food processor or blender, purée soup in batches until smooth. Sprinkle with parsley before serving.

NUTRITIONAL ANALYSIS	Energy	Protein	Carbohydrate	Fat	Iron
per 1/2 cup (125 mL)	76 kcal	4.9 g	11.0 g	1.5 g	1.09 mg

12 to 18 months

Makes 4 cups (1 L)

Tomato Minestrone

*Most versions of minestrone – Italy's national soup –
contain tomatoes, macaroni and, frequently, beans. This version
features plenty of vegetables and macaroni, but no beans.*

Kitchen Tips

Beef stock can be replaced by an equal quantity of canned beef broth, or water mixed with beef bouillon cubes or sachets.

For younger children, this soup can be puréed (or pressed through a sieve) to give it a smoother, thicker consistency.

1 tsp	olive oil	5 mL
1/2 cup	finely chopped onions	125 mL
1	small carrot, chopped	1
1	small zucchini, chopped	1
1	stalk celery, sliced	1
1 cup	diced tomatoes	250 mL
1	clove garlic, minced	1
3 cups	beef stock (see Tip)	750 mL
1/4 tsp	dried basil	1 mL
1/4 tsp	dried oregano	1 mL
1/4 tsp	salt	1 mL
1/4 cup	macaroni	50 mL
	Grated Parmesan cheese, optional	

1. In a large saucepan, heat oil over medium heat. Add onions and cook for 5 minutes or until softened. Add carrot, zucchini, celery, tomatoes, garlic, broth, basil, oregano and salt. Cover and bring to a boil. Reduce heat and simmer for about 15 minutes.

2. Add macaroni and cook for 10 minutes or until macaroni is tender. Serve sprinkled with Parmesan, if using.

NUTRITIONAL ANALYSIS	Energy	Protein	Carbohydrate	Fat	Iron
per 1/2 cup (125 mL)	51 kcal	2.5 g	8.5 g	1.0 g	0.57 mg

12 to 18 months

Makes 6 1/2 cups (1.625 L)

Serves 8

Apple and Butternut Squash Soup

Kitchen Tip

Serve with hot bread or buns.

4 cups	chicken stock	1 L
1	medium butternut squash, peeled, seeded and cut into 2-inch (5 cm) cubes	1
2	medium tart apples, peeled, cored and sliced	2
1 1/4 cups	chopped onions	300 mL
1 tsp	salt	5 mL
1/2 tsp	freshly ground black pepper	2 mL
1/2 tsp	dried rosemary	2 mL
1/2 tsp	dried thyme	2 mL
1/4 cup	light (10%) cream	50 mL

1. In a large pot, combine stock, squash, apples, onions, salt, pepper, rosemary and thyme. Bring to a boil. Reduce heat and simmer for 15 minutes or until vegetables are tender. Remove from heat and stir in cream. Allow soup to cool slightly

2. In a food processor or blender, purée soup in batches until smooth, transferring each batch to a saucepan. Bring to a boil before serving.

NUTRITIONAL ANALYSIS	Energy	Protein	Carbohydrate	Fat	Iron
per 1/2 cup (125 mL)	70 kcal	2.6 g	10.8 g	2.3 g	0.79 mg

12 to 18 months

Serves 6

Makes 4 cups (1 L)

Split-Pea Soup

Enjoy this easy-to-prepare soup on cold days.
The aroma and flavors are classic.

Kitchen Tip

Depending on the age of your child, you can purée this soup or serve it as is. Because it cooks for so long, the soup has a very smooth, thick consistency, with just a few tender chunks.

1 cup	dried split peas, washed	250 mL
6 cups	water	1.5 L
1 cup	finely chopped ham or 4 slices bacon, diced	250 mL
1	medium onion, chopped	1
1	stalk celery, chopped	1
1	medium carrot, peeled and chopped	1
	Salt and freshly ground black pepper to taste	

1. In a large saucepan, combine peas, water, ham, onion, celery and carrot. Bring to a boil; reduce heat to low and simmer for 2 hours or until vegetables and peas are tender. Remove from heat and allow to cool slightly.

2. In a food processor or blender, purée soup in batches until smooth (see Tip). Season to taste with salt and pepper before serving.

NUTRITIONAL ANALYSIS	Energy	Protein	Carbohydrate	Fat	Iron
per 1/2 cup (125 mL)	134 kcal	10.0 g	19.0 g	2.3 g	1.52 mg

12 to 18 months

Makes 8 cups (2 L)

Beef Barley Soup

Kitchen Tips

This soup is great for preparing in a slow cooker. Just add all ingredients and cook on HIGH for 8 to 10 hours or LOW for 10 to 12 hours.

Beef stock can be replaced with canned beef stock or bouillon cubes; in this case you may not need additional salt.

1/4 cup	pearl barley	50 mL
6 cups	beef stock or bouillon, divided	1.5 L
2 tbsp	butter *or* margarine	25 mL
1	onion, chopped	1
2	carrots, chopped	2
Half	turnip, chopped	Half
1	stalk celery, chopped	1
2 cups	diced cooked stewing beef	500 mL
	Salt and freshly ground black pepper to taste	

1. In a large pot, combine barley with 3 cups (750 mL) of the beef stock. Simmer over low heat for 1 1/2 to 2 hours. Add butter.

2. In a saucepan combine vegetables and remaining beef stock. Cook over medium heat for 20 minutes or until tender. Pour vegetables and stock into pot with barley mixture. Season to taste with the salt and pepper. Add cooked meat just before serving.

NUTRITIONAL ANALYSIS	Energy	Protein	Carbohydrate	Fat	Iron
per 1/2 cup (125 mL)	74 kcal	7.4 g	3.9 g	3.1 g	0.94 mg

12 to 18 months

Makes 7 cups (1.75 L)

Chicken Rice Soup

Kitchen Tip

This recipe is easily converted into chicken noodle soup by omitting the rice and adding 1 1/2 cups (375) cooked egg noodles.

5 cups	chicken stock	1.25 L
1/4 cup	chopped onion	50 mL
1/2 cup	chopped celery	125 mL
1/2 cup	chopped carrots	125 mL
3/4 tsp	salt	4 mL
1/8 tsp	freshly ground black pepper	0.5 mL
1 cup	chopped cooked chicken	250 mL
3 tbsp	long grain rice	50 mL

1. In a large pot, combine stock. onion, celery, carrots, salt and pepper. Bring to a boil. Reduce heat and simmer until the vegetables are tender. Add rice and cook for about 15 minutes or until tender. Add cooked chicken and simmer for another 5 minutes.

NUTRITIONAL ANALYSIS per 1/2 cup (125 mL)	Energy	Protein	Carbohydrate	Fat	Iron
	42 kcal	4.9 g	3.3 g	0.8 g	0.37 mg

12 to 18 months

Makes 7 cups (1.75 L)

Cauliflower Soup

1 tbsp	butter *or* margarine	15 mL
8 oz	cauliflower, chopped	250 g
2	onions, chopped	2
4	stalks celery, chopped	4
3 tbsp	all-purpose flour	45 mL
4 cups	chicken stock or vegetable stock	1L
1	bay leaf	1
	Salt and freshly ground black pepper to taste	
2/3 cup	milk or cream	150 mL
1 tbsp	chopped parsley	15 mL

1. In a large saucepan, melt butter over medium heat. Add vegetables and cook for 2 minutes. Do NOT brown. Stir in flour and cook for another minute. Remove from heat. Add stock, bay leaf, salt and pepper. Simmer for about 1 hour until vegetables are tender. Remove and discard bay leaf.

2. Serve soup as is or transfer in batches to a food processor and process until smooth. Add milk and parsley. Reheat and serve.

NUTRITIONAL ANALYSIS	Energy	Protein	Carbohydrate	Fat	Iron
per 1/2 cup (125 mL)	39 kcal	2.5 g	4.0 g	1.5 g	0.43 mg

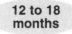

12 to 18 months

Makes 4 cups (1 L)

Sandwich 'n' Soup in a Bowl

Kitchen Tips

If you prefer, the soup can be cooked in the microwave oven on High for about 5 minutes; stir once. Allow to cool, checking temperature before serving to infants.

Save any leftovers for another meal.

This easy-to-prepare vegetarian soup is made from ingredients usually found in your kitchen cupboard.

1	can (14 oz [398 mL]) diced tomatoes	1
1	can (14 oz [398 mL]) beans in tomato sauce	1
3/4 cup	water	175 mL
1/2 tsp	dried basil	2 mL
1/2 tsp	dried oregano	2 mL
1/8 tsp	salt	0.5 mL
1/8 tsp	freshly ground black pepper	0.5 mL
4	slices whole wheat or white bread	4
1/2 cup	shredded mozzarella cheese	125 mL

1. In a large saucepan, combine tomatoes, beans, water, basil, oregano and salt. Bring to a boil. Reduce heat to low and simmer, covered, for 10 minutes. (Soup can also be cooked in microwave; see Tip.)

2. Meanwhile, toast bread. Cut each slice into cubes.

3. Spoon 1 cup (250 mL) soup into each bowl (or about 1/4 cup [50 mL] for an infant's portion). Garnish with bread cubes and sprinkle with cheese. For larger portions, microwave bowls for a few seconds on High or until cheese melts. Infant portions need not be heated; cheese will melt from the heat of the soup as it cools to a baby-friendly serving temperature.

NUTRITIONAL ANALYSIS per 1/2 cup (125 mL)	Energy	Protein	Carbohydrate	Fat	Iron
	139 kcal	8.5 g	21.0 g	3.5 g	0.91 mg

12 to 18 months

Cock-a-Leekie Soup

Makes 7 cups (1.75 L)

Kitchen Tips

For a hearty, chunky soup, serve without puréeing.

If you'd prefer a clearer soup, replace milk with additional chicken stock.

1 tbsp	butter or margarine	15 mL
3	leeks, washed and sliced	3
1 1/2 tbsp	all-purpose flour	22 mL
1 lb	potatoes, peeled and chopped	500 g
2 or 3	stalks celery, chopped	2 or 3
2 1/2 cups	chicken stock	625 mL
1	bay leaf	1
	Salt and freshly ground black pepper to taste	
1 1/4 cups	milk or cream	300 mL
1 tbsp	chopped parsley	15 mL

1. In a large saucepan, melt butter over medium heat. Add leeks and cook for 1 minute. Add flour and cook for another minute. Stir in potatoes and celery. Add chicken stock, bay leaf, salt and pepper. Simmer for 1 hour or until vegetables are very tender. Remove and discard bay leaf.

2. Transfer soup in batches to a food processor and process until smooth. (Alternatively, you can mash the solids by hand). Add milk and parsley. Reheat and serve.

NUTRITIONAL ANALYSIS	Energy	Protein	Carbohydrate	Fat	Iron
per 1/2 cup (125 mL)	77 kcal	2.9 g	13.1 g	1.7 g	0.89 mg

12 to 18 months

Serves 4

Devilled Eggs

Devilled eggs are a favorite with all ages – particularly infants. The eggs are somewhat "squishy" when held in small hands (which is half the fun), and the messy fingers are great for licking.

Kitchen Tip

If you or your family don't care for cottage cheese, omit it and use extra mayonnaise.

To hard-cook eggs: Place cold eggs in a single layer in a saucepan. Add enough water to cover eggs by at least 1 inch (2.5 cm). Bring to a full boil. Remove pan from heat, cover and let eggs stand in hot water for 20 to 25 minutes. Run cold water over eggs until they are completely cooled. Hard-cooked eggs, peeled or in their shells, can be refrigerated for up to one week. If peeled, they are best stored in a plastic bag or other airtight plastic container.

Food Safety Tip

Refrigerating prepared eggs will help reduce the risk of food-borne illnesses. Make sure the refrigerator is set to a temperature of 40° F (4° C).

4	hard-cooked eggs, peeled (see Tip)	4
1/2 cup	cottage cheese (see Tip)	125 mL
2 tbsp	mayonnaise	25 mL
1 tbsp	finely diced onion	15 mL
1/4 tsp	salt	1 mL
1/8 tsp	freshly ground black pepper	0.5 mL
1/8 tsp	paprika	0.5 mL

1. Cut each egg in half lengthwise. Remove yolks and transfer to a small bowl; mash together with cottage cheese, mayonnaise and onion. Stir in salt and pepper.

2. Fill egg whites with yolk mixture; sprinkle lightly with paprika. For best flavor, cover and refrigerate for about 1 hour before serving.

NUTRITIONAL ANALYSIS	Energy	Protein	Carbohydrate	Fat	Iron
per half egg	76 kcal	5.0 g	0.9 g	5.8 g	0.58 mg

Makes 32 bites

LUNCH

Salmon Bites

Serve these small quiche-like squares for baby lunches or snacks – or as appetizers for parents.

PREHEAT OVEN TO 350° F (180° C)
8-INCH (2 L) SQUARE BAKING PAN, GREASED

Kitchen Tip

Leave salmon bones in, but mash well before serving to a small child – they're an excellent source of calcium.

Food Safety Tip

Prepare foods quickly, cook them thoroughly and serve immediately. Don't let potentially unsafe foods linger at room temperature, where bacteria can grow quickly.

1 cup	cottage cheese	250 mL
Half	pkg (8 oz [250 g]) cream cheese	Half
3	eggs	3
1 tbsp	lemon juice	15 mL
1/4 tsp	salt	1 mL
1/4 tsp	dried thyme	1 mL
1	can (7.5 oz [213 g]) salmon, drained	1
1/4 cup	finely chopped onion	50 mL

1. In a food processor or blender, combine cottage cheese, cream cheese, eggs, lemon juice, salt and thyme; process until smooth. Transfer mixture to a bowl.

2. In another bowl, flake salmon; mash bones. Stir salmon into cheese-egg mixture. Stir in onion.

3. Spoon mixture into prepared pan. Bake in a preheated oven for 40 minutes or until a knife inserted in center comes out clean. Remove from oven and allow to stand for 5 minutes before cutting into small fingers.

NUTRITIONAL ANALYSIS	Energy	Protein	Carbohydrate	Fat	Iron
per "bite"	41 kcal	3.2 g	0.5 g	2.8 g	0.25 mg

12 to 18 months

Makes 1 3/4 cups (425 mL)

Egg Salad

Kitchen Tip

If your child does not have an allergy, eggs are a great source of protein.

The curry in this recipe is not overwhelming and adds a slightly different twist to an old favorite.

5	hard-boiled eggs, finely chopped	5
Half	small onion, finely chopped	Half
1/4 cup	mayonnaise	50 mL
Dash	curry powder	Dash
Pinch	salt	Pinch
Pinch	freshly ground black pepper	Pinch

1. In a bowl combine all ingredients and mix well. Use for sandwiches or serve filling on its own.

NUTRITIONAL ANALYSIS per 1/4 cup (50 mL)	Energy	Protein	Carbohydrate	Fat	Iron
	106 kcal	4.5 g	1.0 g	9.2 g	0.82 mg

12 to 18 months

Serves 4

Makes 1 cup (250 mL)

Ham Salad Sandwich

Many parents tell us that even the fussiest child can almost always be persuaded to eat a ham sandwich. This variation on the simple slice-of-ham type sandwich, adds a little more interest.

3/4 cup	diced ham	175 mL
1/4 cup	shredded Cheddar cheese	50 mL
1 tbsp	finely minced green onion	15 mL
2 tbsp	mayonnaise	25 mL
2 tbsp	butter or margarine	25 mL
8	slices whole wheat bread, crusts removed if desired	8

1. In a small bowl, stir together ham, cheese, onion and mayonnaise.

2. Thinly spread each bread slice with butter. Spread 4 slices with 1/4 cup (50 mL) filling. Top with remaining slices. Cut each sandwich into 4 squares and serve.

NUTRITIONAL ANALYSIS	Energy	Protein	Carbohydrate	Fat	Iron
per 1/4 cup (50 mL)	142 kcal	7.9 g	11 g	11.6 g	0.37 mg

Serves 1

French Toast Cheese Sandwich

Kitchen Tip

For a change of flavor, try replacing processed Cheddar cheese with Swiss, mozzarella or other cheeses.

Make this quick lunch in the morning when the toaster is out and refrigerate until lunchtime. Then, pop it into the microwave oven for a speedy and tasty lunch.

2	slices whole wheat bread, toasted	2
1	slice processed Cheddar cheese (see Tip)	1
1	egg, lightly beaten	1
2 tbsp	2% milk	25 mL
1/4 tsp	dried basil	1 mL
1/4 tsp	dried thyme	1 mL
1/8 tsp	salt	0.5 mL
1/8 tsp	freshly ground black pepper	0.5 mL

1. Place toast slice in microwaveable pie plate or other shallow pan. Top with cheese slice, then second toast slice.

2. In a small bowl, whisk together egg, milk, basil, thyme, salt and pepper. Pour over sandwich. Cover with plastic wrap and refrigerate for about 2 hours.

3. Lift one corner of plastic wrap to allow steam to escape. Microwave at Medium for 2 minutes; rotate and microwave for another 90 seconds or until sandwiches are cooked through and no longer moist. Cut into small pieces and allow to cool before serving.

NUTRITIONAL ANALYSIS	Energy	Protein	Carbohydrate	Fat	Iron
	332 kcal	18.1 g	33.2 g	15.0 g	3.68 mg

12 to 18 months

LUNCH

Sloppy Joe Sauce

Makes 5 cups (1.25 L)

Kitchen Tip

This versatile sauce is a great source of iron for the whole family. It freezes well and can be quickly thawed and heated for an instant lunch or dinner.

1 lb	ground beef	500 g
1	onion, finely chopped	1
1	can (28 oz [796 mL]) tomatoes, crushed	1
1 tbsp	vinegar	15 mL
2 tsp	brown sugar	10 mL
1 tsp	salt	5 mL
1 tsp	Worcestershire Sauce	5 mL
1 tsp	prepared mustard	5 mL
1 tbsp	ketchup	15 mL
	Hot dog or hamburger buns	

1. In a frying pan over medium-high heat, cook ground beef, breaking up meat with a spoon, until browned. Drain off fat. With a slotted spoon, transfer beef to a paper towel-lined plate or colander to drain.

2. Add onions to frying pan and sauté until soft. Return beef to pan, along with tomatoes, vinegar, brown sugar, salt, Worcestershire sauce, mustard and ketchup. Simmer over low heat, stirring occasionally, for about 45 minutes or until thick.

3. Serve on hot dog or hamburger buns.

NUTRITIONAL ANALYSIS	Energy	Protein	Carbohydrate	Fat	Iron
per 1/2 cup (125 mL)	145 kcal	10.5 g	8.6 g	7.8 g	1.67 mg

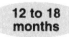
12 to 18 months

Makes 12

Tuna and Corn Patties

Kitchen Tip

This recipe provides an excellent use for corn left over from Corn Chowder (see recipe, page 111).

Food Safety Tip

Make time in your schedule to regularly sanitize countertops, cutting boards and utensils with a mild solution of bleach and water. Gives the kitchen that extra-fresh scent!

Just about everyone has a can of tuna or salmon in their kitchen cupboard. Either works well in these great tasting patties.

1 1/2 cups	biscuit mix	375 mL
1/2 tsp	dried dill	2 mL
1	can (6 1/2 oz [184 g]) tuna, drained and flaked	1
1 cup	cream-style corn	250 mL
1 tbsp	finely chopped onion	15 mL
2	eggs	2
1/2 cup	whole milk	125 mL
2 tsp	vegetable oil, divided	10 mL

1. In a bowl combine biscuit mix and dill. Set aside.

2. In another bowl, combine tuna, corn, onion, eggs and milk; stir to mix well. Stir in biscuit-dill mixture.

3. In a skillet, heat 1 tsp (5 mL) of the oil over medium-high heat. Using a 1/4-cup (50 mL) measure for each patty, drop batter into skillet and cook for about 3 minutes or until bubbles break on surface; turn and cook second side until golden brown. Repeat procedure with remaining batter, adding more oil if needed.

NUTRITIONAL ANALYSIS	Energy	Protein	Carbohydrate	Fat	Iron
per patty	139 kcal	7.4 g	15.7 g	5.3 g	1.06 mg

12 to 18 months

Serves 4 adults or makes 12 baby servings

Carrot 'n' Cheese Crustless Quiche

Kitchen Tip

Zucchini makes a good replacement for carrots in this recipe.

An easy oven luncheon for wintertime, or anytime, this custard combines carrots (some children's favorite vegetable) with eggs and cheese.

PREHEAT OVEN TO 300° F (150° C)

8-INCH (2 L) SQUARE CAKE PAN, GREASED

1 tbsp	butter *or* margarine	15 mL
Half	small onion, finely chopped	Half
1 cup	grated carrots (about 2 medium)	250 mL
1/2 tsp	salt	2 mL
1/2 tsp	curry powder (optional)	2 mL
4	eggs	4
2/3 cup	2% milk	150 mL
1 cup	shredded mozzarella cheese	250 mL
	Paprika	

1. In a skillet, heat butter over medium heat. Add onion and sauté for 5 minutes. Add carrots, salt and curry powder, if using; cook for 5 minutes or until golden brown. Remove from heat; allow to cool.

2. In a medium bowl, whisk together eggs and milk; stir into vegetable mixture. Pour into prepared baking pan. Bake in preheated oven for 20 minutes.

3. Remove quiche from oven. Top with cheese and sprinkle with paprika. Return to oven and bake for another 15 minutes or until custard is firm and cheese is melted. Cut into squares to serve.

NUTRITIONAL ANALYSIS	Energy	Protein	Carbohydrate	Fat	Iron
per baby serving	106 kcal	8.2 g	2.7 g	6.8 g	0.50 mg

Serves 2 adults

Makes 5 baby servings

Macaroni and Vegetables with Cheese

Kitchen Tip

Use leftover cooked vegetables or frozen mixed vegetables, thawed.

*Here's a healthy, vegetable-packed version of classic mac and cheese!
Use any vegetables that appeal to your family. Little ones are
always fascinated by macaroni's squishy texture.*

PREHEAT OVEN TO 350° F (180° C)

3-CUP (750 ML) CASSEROLE, GREASED

3/4 cup	uncooked macaroni	175 mL
2 cups	water	500 mL
1 1/2 cups	shredded medium Cheddar cheese, divided	375 mL
1 tbsp	butter *or* margarine	15 mL
1/2 cup	whole milk	125 mL
3/4 cup	mixed cooked vegetables (such as carrots, peas, corn, broccoli and/or green beans)	175 mL
1/2 cup	coarse whole wheat bread crumbs	125 mL

1. In a medium saucepan, cook macaroni in boiling water according to package directions or until tender but firm). Drain. Add 1 cup (250 mL) of the cheese, butter, milk and vegetables. Stir until cheese is melted.

2. Spoon into prepared casserole; top with crumbs and remaining cheese. Bake in preheated oven for 25 minutes or until crumbs are brown and macaroni is hot.

NUTRITIONAL ANALYSIS	Energy	Protein	Carbohydrate	Fat	Iron
per 1/2 cup (125 mL)	302 kcal	14.1 g	26.6 g	15.4 g	1.15 mg

12 to 18 months

Makes 3 cups (750 mL)

Marinated Vegetables

Crisp raw vegetables gain great flavor – and favor – when marinated in a light dressing of olive oil and vinegar. Junior diners will enjoy eating these veggies alone or with cubes of cheese. Parents may wish to place the vegetables on paper toweling to absorb excess marinade before serving to finger-eaters.

Kitchen Tip

If your child prefers vegetables partially cooked, just blanch them in a saucepan of boiling water for about 2 minutes, then plunge into cold water to stop the cooking.

Food Safety Tip

Refrigerate prepared vegetables or any leftovers within 2 hours after cooking.

1	medium carrot, sliced (see Tip)	1
1/2 cup	frozen peas, thawed	125 mL
1/2 cup	sliced yellow beans	125 mL
1/2 cup	small broccoli florets	125 mL
1/2 cup	small cauliflower florets	125 mL
1/2 cup	tomato juice	125 mL
1 tbsp	olive oil	15 mL
1 tbsp	red wine vinegar	15 mL
1/2 tsp	dried basil	2 mL
1/2 tsp	dried oregano	2 mL
Pinch	salt	Pinch
Pinch	freshly ground black pepper	Pinch

1. Place carrot, peas, beans, broccoli and cauliflower in a plastic bag.

2. In a tightly sealed container, shake together tomato juice, oil, vinegar, basil, oregano, salt and pepper. Add dressing to vegetables; seal bag and shake to distribute evenly. Marinate in the refrigerator for several hours. Drain and serve. Vegetables will keep in the refrigerator for several days.

NUTRITIONAL ANALYSIS	Energy	Protein	Carbohydrate	Fat	Iron
per 1/4 cup (50 mL)	24 kcal	0.8 g	2.8 g	1.2 g	0.36 mg

Makes 2 cups (500 mL)

Vegetables with Cheese

This combination of cheese and vegetables is bound to entice children to eat their vegetables.

1 cup	thinly sliced carrots	250 mL
1 cup	thinly sliced zucchini	250 mL
1/2 cup	processed Cheddar cheese spread	125 mL
2 tbsp	light (10%) cream or milk	25 mL
1/2 tsp	dried basil	2 mL

1. In a small saucepan, combine carrots and zucchini with just enough water to cover. Bring to a boil; cook for 10 minutes or until tender. Drain. Stir in cheese, milk and basil. Return saucepan to low heat; cook until warmed through and cheese melts.

NUTRITIONAL ANALYSIS	Energy	Protein	Carbohydrate	Fat	Iron
per 1/4 cup (50 mL)	51 kcal	2.8 g	3.1 g	3.1 g	0.26 mg

12 to 18 months

Makes 2 cups (500 mL)

Lunchtime Pasta and Bean Casserole

Kitchen Tips

Mixed vegetables are usually a combination of frozen peas, corn, green beans and carrots cut into small pieces.

Any kidney beans and tomato soup leftovers can be used another day to make chili.

A colorful and interesting combination of foods, this casserole is well suited to any finger-eaters in your family. Omit the kidney beans if you wish, but they do provide extra protein and fiber.

1/2 cup	shell pasta	125 mL
1/2 cup	frozen mixed vegetables (see Tip)	125 mL
1/2 cup	canned kidney beans, rinsed and drained (optional)	125 mL
1/4 cup	shredded mozzarella or Cheddar cheese	50 mL
1/4 cup	condensed tomato soup	50 mL
1/4 cup	milk	50 mL
1/8 tsp	salt	0.5 mL
1/8 tsp	freshly ground black pepper	0.5 mL

1. In a medium saucepan, cook pasta in boiling water for 5 minutes until it is just beginning to soften. Add mixed vegetables. Return to a boil and cook until pasta is until tender but firm. Drain well.

2. Add kidney beans, if using, and cheese; stir until cheese has melted. Stir in tomato soup and milk. Season to taste with salt and pepper.

NUTRITIONAL ANALYSIS	Energy	Protein	Carbohydrate	Fat	Iron
per 1/2 cup (125 mL)	156 kcal	8.6 g	23.8 g	3.0 g	1.13 mg

Makes 2 baby servings

Broccoli with Pasta

Kitchen Tip

If you don't have stock, use 1/2 tsp (2 mL) liquid chicken or vegetable bouillon concentrate with enough added water to make 1/4 cup (50 mL).

Variation

Other vegetables can replace (or be added to) broccoli. Try cooked carrots, peas, corn or mixed vegetables.

Cook this up when little appetites can't wait another minute. For fastest preparation, keep cooked broccoli and cooked pasta on hand in the refrigerator. Broccoli's vitamins and minerals, and pasta's protein make this a nutritious meal.

1 tsp	olive oil	5 mL
2 tbsp	finely chopped onion	25 mL
1/4 cup	chicken or vegetable stock (see Tip)	50 mL
1/4 cup	chopped cooked broccoli	50 mL
1/2 cup	cooked macaroni or other pasta	125 mL
1 tsp	grated Parmesan cheese	5 mL

1. In a small skillet, heat oil on medium heat. Add onion and cook for 3 minutes. Add broth, broccoli and pasta; cook, covered, until just heated through. Add cheese; toss and serve.

NUTRITIONAL ANALYSIS	Energy	Protein	Carbohydrate	Fat	Iron
per baby serving	90 kcal	3.5 g	12.0 g	3.2 g	0.51 mg

over 18 months

LUNCH

Macaroni and Cheese

Makes 6 cups (1.5 L)

PREHEAT OVEN TO 375° F (190° C)
8-CUP (2 L) CASSEROLE

Kitchen Tip

Want a lower-fat version of this dish? In Step 2, omit the butter; heat the milk until hot (but not boiling) and add 2 oz (50 g) light cream cheese. Mix flour with grated Cheddar; gradually add it to the milk mixture, stirring until Cheddar cheese has melted and the sauce is thick. Continue with Step 3.

2 1/2 cups	macaroni	625 mL
3 tbsp	butter or margarine	45 mL
1/4 cup	all-purpose flour	50 mL
2 cups	milk	500 mL
2 cups	grated old Cheddar cheese	500 mL
1/4 tsp	dry mustard	2 mL
	Salt and freshly ground black pepper to taste	

Topping

1/2 cup	fine dry bread crumbs	125 mL
1 tbsp	butter or margarine, melted	15 mL
2 tbsp	grated old Cheddar cheese	25 mL
Dash	paprika	Dash

1. In a large saucepan, cook the macaroni according to package instructions or until tender but firm.

2. In another large saucepan, melt butter over medium heat. Add flour and cook, stirring, until it starts to bubble. Gradually add milk, stirring constantly, and cook until thickened. Add grated cheese; stir until melted. Stir in mustard; season to taste with salt and pepper.

3. Transfer drained macaroni to prepared casserole; pour sauce over. Stir just until mixed.

4. Topping: In a bowl combine bread crumbs and melted butter; distribute evenly over macaroni. Sprinkle with 2 tbsp (25 mL) cheese and paprika.

5. Bake in preheated oven for 30 minutes or until mixture is heated through and topping is browned.

NUTRITIONAL ANALYSIS	Energy	Protein	Carbohydrate	Fat	Iron
per 1/2 cup (125 mL)	277 kcal	11.2 g	29.2 g	12.6 g	0.90 mg

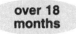

Makes about 6 1/2 cups (1.6 L)

Junior Hot-and-Sour Soup

Kitchen Tip

Start with the lesser quantity of pepper sauce for children who are not be used to spicier food.

So easy and fast to make, yet delicious and tasty.
Adjust the amount of pepper sauce used to individual tastes.
A good way to introduce kids to spicier foods.

6 cups	chicken stock	1.5 L
3 tbsp	soy sauce	45 mL
4 tsp	ground ginger	20 mL
1 tbsp	rice vinegar	15 mL
2 tsp	granulated sugar	10 mL
1/2 to 1 tsp	hot pepper sauce (see Tip)	2 to 5 mL
1 tsp	sesame oil	5 mL
4 oz	silken tofu, diced	125 g
2	green onions, sliced	2

1. In a large saucepan, combine stock with soy sauce, ginger, vinegar, sugar, pepper sauce and sesame oil. Bring to a boil. Add tofu and green onions. Cook for 1 minute longer and serve.

NUTRITIONAL ANALYSIS	Energy	Protein	Carbohydrate	Fat	Iron
per 1/2 cup (125 mL)	37 kcal	3.6 g	2.1 g	1.5 g	0.95 mg

over 18 months

Serves 1

Grilled Fruit 'n' Cheese Sandwich

Layers of fruit and cheese sandwiched between bread supplies three food groups at once. Add a glass of milk for a fast, easy and nutritious lunch that will be enjoyed by all.

2	slices whole wheat bread	2
2	slices processed cheese	2
5	thin slices apple or pear	5
1 tsp	butter *or* margarine	5 mL

1. Place bread slice on cutting board. Place one cheese slice on bread, top with fruit slices, then second cheese slice. Add second bread slice, spread outside of sandwich lightly with butter on both sides.

2. Heat a nonstick skillet over medium heat. Add sandwich, cover and cook for 3 minutes or until underside becomes golden brown. With a spatula, turn sandwich over and cook until second side is browned and cheese starts to melt.

3. Remove to a cutting board and cut sandwich into small finger-like pieces. (Remove crust if appropriate.) Be sure to allow sandwich to cool sufficiently before serving.

NUTRITIONAL ANALYSIS	Energy	Protein	Carbohydrate	Fat	Iron
per sandwich	361 kcal	16.4 g	33.6 g	19.2 g	2.01 mg

Serves 4
Makes 8 wedges

Mexican Quesadilla Sandwich

In Spanish, queso *means cheese. Combine it with a tortilla, you end up with a quesadilla. This dish is ideal for young ones – small enough to clutch easily, and the filling keeps the tortillas from falling apart.*

2	9-inch (22.5 cm) flour tortillas	2
1/2 tbsp	salsa or ketchup	7 mL
1/4 cup	shredded Cheddar cheese	50 mL
1/4 cup	canned beans in tomato sauce, mashed	50 mL

1. Place 1 tortilla on a microwaveable plate lined with paper towels. Spread with salsa.

2. In a small bowl, combine cheese and beans. Spoon mixture evenly over tortilla. Press second tortilla over bean mixture.

3. Microwave at Medium-High for 2 minutes or until tortillas are warm and cheese has melted. (For a crisper tortilla, bake in a preheated 350° F (180° C) oven for 10 minutes.) With sharp knife, cut into 8 small pie-shaped pieces. Allow to cool before serving.

NUTRITIONAL ANALYSIS	Energy	Protein	Carbohydrate	Fat	Iron
per wedge	50 kcal	2.0 g	6.2 g	2.0 g	0.22 mg

over 18
months

LUNCH

Ham and Cheese Melt

Serves 1

*Make a slice of ham and cheese into something different
than "just another sandwich".*

PREHEAT BROILER
BAKING SHEET

Variation

Replace ham with flaked tuna or
salmon. Combine fish, cheese
and mayonnaise. Spread on each
bread slice and broil as directed
in recipe.

1/4 cup	diced cooked ham	50 mL
1/4 cup	shredded Cheddar cheese	50 mL
1 tsp	mayonnaise	5 mL
1	slice whole wheat or multigrain bread	1

1. In a bowl, combine ham, cheese and mayonnaise.
   Spread mixture on bread. Transfer bread to baking
   sheet. Broil just until cheese starts to melt.
   Remove from heat and allow to cool. Cut into
   small pieces before serving.

NUTRITIONAL ANALYSIS	Energy	Protein	Carbohydrate	Fat	Iron
	252 kcal	13.8 g	15.4 g	15.4 g	1.33 mg

over 18
months

Makes 8

Turkey Pita Wedges

Kitchen Tip

Be careful when microwaving
food for young children. It can
quickly become hot enough to
burn their sensitive mouths.

1 cup	shredded Cheddar cheese	250 mL
1 cup	chopped cooked turkey or chicken	250 mL
Half	red bell pepper, cored and thinly sliced	Half
2	pita breads, quartered	2

1. In a small bowl, combine cheese, turkey and red
   pepper. Stuff each pita quarter with turkey mixture. Microwave on High for 30 seconds or until
   the cheese melts. Repeat procedure with remaining quarters. Serve immediately.

NUTRITIONAL ANALYSIS	Energy	Protein	Carbohydrate	Fat	Iron
per wedge	113 kcal	10.4 g	6.6 g	5.1 g	0.40 mg

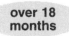

Makes 16

Broccoli and Chicken Pita Pockets

Kitchen Tip

Instead of pita bread, serve filling on a bed of lettuce.

1	medium head broccoli, florets cut into bite-size pieces	1
2 cups	diced cooked chicken	500 mL
1/4 cup	diced celery	50 mL
1/4 cup	diced radishes	50 mL
1/3 cup	mayonnaise	75 mL
1/4 cup	plain yogurt	50 mL
1 tsp	Dijon mustard	5 mL
1/4 tsp	dried rosemary, crushed	1 mL
Dash	salt	Dash
4	pita breads, quartered	4

1. In a large saucepan, blanch the broccoli in boiling water for 1 minute. Drain and rinse under cold water. Drain again.

2. In a large bowl, combine broccoli, chicken, celery and radishes. Set aside.

3. In another large bowl, combine mayonnaise, yogurt, mustard, rosemary and salt. Stir in broccoli mixture. Cover and chill for 1 hour.

4. Spoon the chilled mixture into the pita pieces.

NUTRITIONAL ANALYSIS	Energy	Protein	Carbohydrate	Fat	Iron
per pocket	108 kcal	7.9 g	10.2 g	4.3 g	0.30 mg

over 18 months

Serves 6 adults

Makes 12 baby servings

Cheddar 'n' Apple Quiche

Quiches are a great way to add protein, milk, and fruit or vegetables to a meal. This version is popular with both infants and adults.

PREHEAT OVEN TO 350° F (180° C)

9-INCH (23 CM) PIE PLATE

2 tbsp	butter *or* margarine	25 mL
1 tbsp	finely chopped onion	15 mL
1 cup	coarsely crushed cornflakes	250 mL
2	large apples, peeled, cored and sliced	2
3	eggs	3
1 cup	cottage cheese	250 mL
1 cup	shredded Cheddar cheese	250 mL
1/4 cup	2% milk	50 mL
1/2 tsp	salt	2 mL
1/8 tsp	freshly ground black pepper	0.5 mL
1/8 tsp	ground nutmeg	0.5 mL

1. In a nonstick skillet, melt butter over medium heat. Add onions and cook for 5 minutes or until tender. Stir in cornflakes. Press mixture into pie plate, forming a crust. Bake in preheated oven for 8 minutes.

2. Meanwhile, cook apples in 2 tbsp (25 mL) boiling water for 4 minutes or until barely tender; drain well. Arrange apples in crust.

3. In a blender or food processor, combine eggs, cottage cheese, Cheddar cheese, milk, salt and pepper; process until smooth. Pour into crust. Sprinkle with nutmeg.

4. Bake in preheated oven for 45 minutes or until a knife inserted in center comes out clean. Let stand for 10 minutes before cutting into wedges.

NUTRITIONAL ANALYSIS	Energy	Protein	Carbohydrate	Fat	Iron
per baby serving	118 kcal	6.8 g	6.3 g	7.4 g	0.67 mg

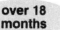

over 18 months

Serves 2

Vegetable Burritos

Kitchen Tip

You may want to cut each burrito into smaller pieces for your toddler.

These burritos are ready in minutes from the microwave oven – the perfect fast fix for a last-minute lunch or dinner.

1	plum tomato, chopped	1
1	small carrot, peeled and thinly sliced	1
4	strips green pepper	4
1/2 cup	refried beans, divided	125 mL
2	8-inch (20 cm) flour tortillas	2
1/2 cup	shredded mozzarella or Cheddar cheese, divided	125 mL
1/8 tsp	dried basil	0.5 mL
1/8 tsp	dried oregano	0.5 mL

1. In a microwavable container, combine tomato, carrot and green pepper. Cover and microwave on High for 2 minutes or until vegetables are tender.

2. Spoon 1/4 cup (50 mL) beans down the center of each tortilla; top with some of the vegetable mixture and 1/4 cup (50 mL) cheese. Fold sides of tortillas into the center. Fold bottom over filling and roll up. Place on a microwavable dish. Microwave at Medium-High for 5 minutes or until burritos are warm (see Tip). Allow to cool to a safe temperature before serving to children.

NUTRITIONAL ANALYSIS	Energy	Protein	Carbohydrate	Fat	Iron
per half burrito	183 kcal	12.0 g	17.8 g	7.2 g	1.35 mg

Makes 1 1/4 cups (300 mL) filling

Falafel-Style Pitas

This smooth chickpea mixture makes a delicious filling for pita breads. Use miniature pitas for little people – they are easier for small hands to hold. The rather sticky filling holds the pita together, much like peanut butter.

Kitchen Tips

Try adding garnishes to the top of the filled pita – such as chopped tomato, green pepper, shredded lettuce.

Keep any leftover filling in the refrigerator for nutritious snacks. It will keep for several days.

Food Safety Tip

Be careful about spreading the filling too thick when serving to young children. Like peanut butter, it should be spread thinly to prevent choking.

1 tsp	olive oil	5 mL
Half	small onion, finely chopped	Half
1	clove garlic, minced	1
1 tbsp	sesame seeds	15 mL
1 cup	chickpeas, rinsed and drained	250 mL
1/2 cup	plain yogurt	125 mL
1/8 tsp	ground cumin	0.5 mL
1/8 tsp	salt	0.5 mL
1/8 tsp	freshly ground black pepper	0.5 mL
2 1/2	whole wheat pita breads (or use miniature pitas)	2 1/2
2 tbsp	shredded mild Cheddar cheese	25 mL

1. In a nonstick skillet, heat oil over medium heat. Add onion, garlic and sesame seeds; cook for 4 minutes or until onion is tender. Allow to cool slightly.

2. In a food processor, combine onion mixture, chickpeas, yogurt, cumin, salt and pepper; process until smooth.

3. Cut regular-sized pitas into halves. Spoon a small amount of mixture into each half and top with a little cheese. (If using miniature pitas, open one side and spoon about 1 tbsp (15 mL) filling into each.)

4. Place each pita on a paper towel-lined microwavable plate; microwave at High for 10 seconds (for miniature pitas) or 30 seconds (for regular size), until cheese has just melted.

NUTRITIONAL ANALYSIS	Energy	Protein	Carbohydrate	Fat	Iron
per 1/4 pita	97 kcal	4.2 g	14.9 g	2.3 g	1.07 mg

over 18 months

Serves 3

Pizza Omelette

Kitchen Tip

Use whatever pizza toppings your kids like. Mozzarella can be replaced by whatever cheese you have in your refrigerator. Cheddar or marble cheese works just as well.

3	eggs	3
2 tbsp	2% milk	25 mL
Pinch	salt	Pinch
Pinch	freshly ground black pepper	Pinch
Pinch	dried basil	Pinch
Pinch	dried oregano	Pinch
1 tbsp	butter *or* margarine	15 mL
2 tbsp	tomato sauce	25 mL
1/4 cup	grated mozzarella cheese	50 mL
1/4 cup	chopped vegetables (such as peppers, mushrooms, etc.)	50 mL

1. In a bowl whisk together eggs, milk, salt, pepper, basil and oregano.

2. In a small skillet with an ovenproof handle, melt butter over medium heat. Add egg mixture and cook until underside is set. With a spatula, flip omelet and cook other side. Garnish with tomato sauce, cheese and vegetables. Place under pre-heated broiler and broil for 1 to 2 minutes until cheese melts.

NUTRITIONAL ANALYSIS	Energy	Protein	Carbohydrate	Fat	Iron
per serving	171 kcal	11.2 g	2.9 g	12.7 g	1.41 mg

Potato Salad

over 18 months

Makes 4 cups (1 L)

Kitchen Tip

For an attractive presentation, garnish with sliced hard-boiled eggs and a dash of paprika.

6	potatoes (preferably a waxy variety), peeled and cut into pieces	6
3/4 cup	mayonnaise	175 mL
1	small onion, chopped	1
2	radishes, chopped	2
1 tsp	prepared mustard	5 mL
1/4 tsp	curry powder	1 mL
	Salt and freshly ground black pepper to taste	

1. In a large saucepan, boil potatoes in water to cover for 15 to 20 minutes, until they are just cooked. Drain and allow to cool. Cut into bite-size pieces.

2. In a large bowl, combine mayonnaise, onion, radishes, mustard, curry powder, salt and pepper. Add potatoes and toss to coat. Chill before serving

NUTRITIONAL ANALYSIS	Energy	Protein	Carbohydrate	Fat	Iron
per 1/4 cup (50 mL)	118 kcal	1.1 g	10.5 g	8.1 g	0.20 mg

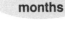

Serves 1

Food Safety Tip

Food served on skewers is considered unsafe for children under 4 years of age. Be sure to remove skewers from kebabs in this recipe.

Children's Cheese Kebabs

PREHEAT BROILER

3	1/2-inch (1 cm) cubes Cheddar cheese	3
3	cherry tomatoes	3
Half	slice bread, buttered and cut into small squares	Half
1	slice bacon, cooked	1

1. On a wooden or metal skewer, place alternating pieces of cheese, tomato, buttered bread and bacon. Place kebab on foil and cook under preheated broiler for 3 minutes, turning once. Remove skewer before serving.

NUTRITIONAL ANALYSIS	Energy	Protein	Carbohydrate	Fat	Iron
	169 kcal	7.6 g	9.2 g	11.4 g	0.78 mg

over 18 months

Serves 2

Kitchen Tip

Use the toppings suggested here – or whatever your child likes best.

English Muffin Mini Pizzas

PREHEAT OVEN TO 350° F (180° C)
BAKING SHEET

1	English muffin, halved	1
1/4 cup	spaghetti sauce	50 mL
1/4 cup	shredded mozzarella cheese	50 mL
6	slices pepperoni	6
2	mushrooms, sliced	2

1. On each half of muffin, divide sauce and the cheese equally. Top each with 3 slices of pepperoni and 1 sliced mushroom. Bake in preheated oven for 10 to 15 minutes or until cheese has melted.

NUTRITIONAL ANALYSIS	Energy	Protein	Carbohydrate	Fat	Iron
per serving	286 kcal	15.2 g	21.4 g	15.4 g	1.62 mg

Dinner

A B C D E F G H I J K L M N O P Q R S T U V W X Y Z

recipe listing continues next page...

Dinner
(continued)

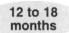

8 to 12 months

Serves 2 or 3

Puréed Baby Meat

1/2 cup	cooked meat (chicken, beef, etc.), cut into small pieces	125 mL
1/4 cup	water *or* cooking liquid *or* milk	50 mL

1. In a food processor or blender, combine meat and water. Process for 1 to 2 minutes or until smooth. Serve immediately or freeze in an ice cube tray for future use.

NUTRITIONAL ANALYSIS	Energy	Protein	Carbohydrate	Fat	Iron
for chicken	115 kcal	21.7 g	0.0 g	2.5 g	0.73 mg
for beef	146 kcal	19.3 g	0.0 g	7.0 g	2,56 mg
for lamb	132 kcal	19,7 g	0.0 g	5.3 g	1.40 mg

12 to 18 months

Serves 4 adults
Makes 8 baby servings

Baked Squash

PREHEAT OVEN TO 350° F (180° C)
SHALLOW BAKING DISH, GREASED

Kitchen Tips

Use whatever variety of squash you like – acorn, buttercup or butternut will work equally well.

Squash is a great source of vitamin A.

1 lb	squash, peeled and sliced	500 g
1	large baking apple, peeled, cored and cut into 1/2-inch [1 cm] rings)	1
1/4 cup	packed brown sugar	50 mL
2 tbsp	margarine	25 mL
1 1/2 tsp	all-purpose flour	7 mL
1/2 tsp	salt	2 mL

1. Arrange squash in prepared baking dish. Top with the apple rings.

2. In a bowl combine brown sugar, margarine, flour and salt. Spread mixture evenly over squash and apples. Bake in preheated oven for 1 nour or until tender.

NUTRITIONAL ANALYSIS	Energy	Protein	Carbohydrate	Fat	Iron
per baby serving	92 kcal	0.7 g	17.1 g	3.0 g	0.67 mg

12 to 18 months

Makes 2 cups (500 mL)

Creamed Spinach

Kitchen Tip

If you wish, omit the bacon and use 1 tbsp (15 mL) olive oil to sauté the onions and garlic.

The recipe may be made ahead and reheated at serving time.

Here's a recipe that raises spinach to new heights of flavor. Many guests who have tasted this vegetable dish request the recipe – especially the mothers of toddlers! It's a great way to get them to eat their spinach.

2	slices bacon, finely chopped (see Tip)	2
1	small onion, finely chopped	1
1	clove garlic, minced	1
2 tbsp	all-purpose flour	25 mL
1/2 tsp	paprika	2 mL
1/2 tsp	salt	2 mL
1/8 tsp	freshly ground black pepper	0.5 mL
1 cup	2% milk	250 mL
1	pkg (10 oz [300 g]) frozen chopped spinach, thawed, excess liquid squeezed out	1

1. In a skillet over medium-high heat, sauté bacon and onion for 5 minutes. Add garlic and cook for 5 minutes or until onions are tender and bacon has become crisp. Remove from heat.

2. Stir in flour paprika, salt and pepper; blend well. Return skillet to heat. Slowly add milk and cook, stirring frequently, until thickened. Stir in spinach, mix well and serve.

NUTRITIONAL ANALYSIS	Energy	Protein	Carbohydrate	Fat	Iron
per 1/4 cup (50 mL)	44 kcal	3.0 g	5.1 g	1.6 g	0.94 mg

12 to 18
months

Serves 1 to 2 adults

Makes 4 baby servings

Baked Sweet Potato

PREHEAT OVEN TO 350° F (180° C)

BAKING SHEET

Kitchen Tip

For infants who may not be able to chew it well, remove skin before serving.

Sweet potatoes are a great source of vitamin A.

1	sweet potato, well scrubbed	1
1 tbsp	butter *or* margarine	15 mL
1 tbsp	maple syrup	15 mL

1. Cut sweet potato into slices 1/2 inch (1 cm) thick and place on baking sheet. Dab a small amount of butter on each slice. Bake in preheated oven for 50 minutes. Remove from oven and drizzle with maple syrup. Bake for another 10 minutes or until tender.

NUTRITIONAL ANALYSIS	Energy	Protein	Carbohydrate	Fat	Iron
per baby serving	72 kcal	0.6 g	11.1 g	3.0 g	0.26 mg

12 to 18
months

Makes 2 1/2 cups (625 mL)

Cucumber Yogurt Dip

This is a thinner, lower-fat version of the famous Greek tzaziki sauce!

2 cups	plain yogurt	500 mL
Half	medium cucumber, peeled and finely chopped	Half
1	clove garlic, minced	1
1 tsp	dried dill	5 mL

1. In a bowl combine yogurt, cucumber, garlic and dill. Refrigerate for at least 1 hour to allow flavors to blend. Serve on a pita or as a side dish with meat.

NUTRITIONAL ANALYSIS	Energy	Protein	Carbohydrate	Fat	Iron
per 1/4 cup (50 mL)	34 kcal	1.9 g	3.0 g	1.7 g	0.12 mg

DINNER

Potato Logs

Kitchen Tip

Instead of cooking potatoes for this recipe, you can use leftover cooked potatoes. Or you can cook extra potatoes and use them for another day's potato logs.

These potato logs freeze well.

With their crunchy coating of cornflake crumbs, these logs make a nice change from plain old mashed potatoes. Children like them not only for their flavor, but for their shape, which is more interesting and less imposing than a glob of ordinary mashed.

PREHEAT OVEN TO 450° F (230° C)

BAKING SHEET, GREASED

3	large potatoes, peeled and cubed	3
2 tbsp	butter *or* margarine	25 mL
1	small onion, finely chopped	1
1/4 cup	whole milk	50 mL
1	egg, beaten	1
1/4 tsp	ground nutmeg	1 mL
1/4 tsp	salt	1 mL
1/4 tsp	freshly ground black pepper	1 mL
3/4 cup	crushed cornflake crumbs	175 mL

1. In a medium saucepan, cook potatoes in boiling water for 15 minutes or until tender. Drain well. Dry drained potatoes over low heat, while shaking pan. Mash potatoes well. Stir in butter, onion, milk, egg, nutmeg, salt and pepper. Beat with an electric mixer until smooth.

2. When mixture is cool enough to handle, shape into small logs. Roll in crushed crumbs and place on prepared baking sheet. Bake in preheated oven for 15 minutes or until browned, turning halfway through baking time.

NUTRITIONAL ANALYSIS	Energy	Protein	Carbohydrate	Fat	Iron
per log	191 kcal	4.6 g	28.8 g	6.7 g	1.27 mg

Serves 4 adults

Makes 12 baby servings

Scalloped Potatoes

This dish is always a family favorite,
especially served with ham or roast pork.

Variation

Add 1/2 cup (125 mL) shredded Cheddar cheese between potato layers.

PREHEAT OVEN TO 350° F (180° C)

4-CUP (1 L) CASSEROLE, GREASED

3 cups	thinly sliced peeled potatoes	750 mL
1	medium onion, chopped	1
2 tbsp	all-purpose flour	25 mL
3 tbsp	butter *or* margarine	45 mL
1 1/4 cups	whole milk	300 mL
1/2 tsp	salt	2 mL
1/4 tsp	freshly ground black pepper	1 mL
1/4 tsp	paprika	1 mL

1. In prepared casserole, alternate layers of potato slices, onions and flour.

2. In a small saucepan, heat butter and milk over low heat until melted; stir in salt and pepper. Pour over layers. Sprinkle with paprika. Bake in preheated oven for 50 minutes or until tender.

NUTRITIONAL ANALYSIS	Energy	Protein	Carbohydrate	Fat	Iron
per baby serving	80 kcal	1.8 g	10.6 g	3.5 g	0.22 mg

12 to 18 months

Serves 2

Garlic Mashed Potato

Kitchen Tip

Potato skins are a great source of fiber.

1	potato (new or red), well scrubbed	1
1	clove garlic	1
1 tsp	butter *or* margarine	5 mL
2 tbsp	2% milk	25 mL

1. Leaving skin on, cut potato into chunks.

2. In a small saucepan, boil potato and garlic for 15 to 20 minutes or until potato is soft. Drain. Add butter and milk. Mash.

NUTRITIONAL ANALYSIS	Energy	Protein	Carbohydrate	Fat	Iron
per serving	85 kcal	1.8 g	14.8 g	2.3 g	0.25 mg

12 to 18 months

Makes 6 cups (1.5 L)

Super Simple Hash Browns

PREHEAT OVEN TO 350° F (180° C)

8-CUP (2 L) CASSEROLE

1	bag (1 lb [454 g]) frozen hash brown potatoes	1
1/2 cup	sour cream	125 mL
1 1/2 cups	grated Cheddar cheese	375 mL
1	can (10 oz [284 mL]) cream of mushroom soup	1
1/2 cup	butter *or* margarine	125 mL

1. In a large bowl, combine hash browns, sour cream, cheese, soup and butter; mix well. Transfer mixture to casserole. Bake for about 1 1/2 hours or until golden brown.

NUTRITIONAL ANALYSIS	Energy	Protein	Carbohydrate	Fat	Iron
per 1/4 cup (50 mL)	102 kcal	2.6 g	4.6 g	8.3 g	0.30 mg

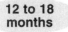
Serves 4 adults

Makes 8 baby servings

Mashed Potato Casserole

Kitchen Tip

Sour cream is a good replacement for milk.

This dish is a favorite with the young set, who all seem to love mashed potatoes. Anytime you have leftover mashed potatoes, use them in this recipe.

PREHEAT OVEN TO 400° F (200° C)

4-CUP (1 L) CASSEROLE, GREASED

3	large potatoes, peeled and cubed	3
1/4 cup	2% milk (see Tip)	50 mL
1/4 tsp	ground nutmeg	1 mL
1/4 tsp	salt	1 mL
1/4 tsp	freshly ground black pepper	1 mL
2 tbsp	butter or margarine	25 mL
Half	small onion, finely chopped	Half
1/4 cup	dry bread crumbs	50 mL
1 tbsp	melted butter or margarine	15 mL

1. In a large saucepan, cook potatoes in boiling water for 20 minutes or until tender. Drain well; dry potatoes over low heat. Mash potatoes. Stir in milk, nutmeg, salt and pepper.

2. In a small skillet, melt butter. Add onion and sauté for 5 minutes or until softened. Stir into potatoes.

3. Spoon potatoes into prepared casserole. Combine bread crumbs with 1 tbsp (15 mL) of the melted butter. Sprinkle over potatoes. Bake in a preheated oven for 20 minutes or until heated through and crumbs are golden brown.

NUTRITIONAL ANALYSIS	Energy	Protein	Carbohydrate	Fat	Iron
per baby serving	93 kcal	1.6 g	12.7 g	4.2 g	0.25 mg

12 to 18 months

Makes 3 cups (750 mL)

Classic Creamy Risotto

This traditional Italian rice dish is a favorite with young children.
They love its creaminess, cheese flavor and soft texture.
Their parents love it for the same reasons.

Risotto Tips

Arborio rice is much easier to find in supermarkets today, thanks to the growing popularity of risotto.

There are several easy but important steps in cooking risotto.

* Keep the broth hot.

* Allow all the liquid to be absorbed before more stock is added. This results in rice with a creamy texture while the grains remain separate and firm.

* Contrary to popular belief, it is unnecessary to stir risotto constantly. All that's required is an occasional stir as you pass by the stove, keeping the mixture at a slow boil.

* For a traditional flavor for adults, add 1/4 cup (50 mL) white wine in Step 2 as a replacement for the same amount of stock. It should be added before any broth to increase the flavor of the dish.

Variations

While rice is cooking, sauté assorted chopped vegetables in oil until soft, then stir them into the cooked risotto just before serving. Try mushrooms, red or yellow bell peppers or zucchini.

Other foods you can add to risotto include cooked vegetables, shellfish, chicken, beef, sausage, as well as other cheeses and herbs.

2 tsp	olive oil	10 mL
2 tsp	butter *or* margarine	10 mL
1/4 cup	finely chopped onion	50 mL
1	clove garlic, minced	1
1 cup	Arborio rice (see Tips)	250 mL
3 cups	hot chicken or vegetable stock	750 mL
1/4 cup	freshly grated Parmesan cheese	50 mL
1/8 tsp	freshly ground black pepper	0.5 mL
1/8 tsp	ground nutmeg	0.5 mL

1. In a large saucepan, heat oil and butter over medium heat. Add onion and garlic; cook for 5 minutes or until tender. Stir in rice and cook for 3 minutes, being careful not to let it brown.

2. Add hot stock, 1/2 cup (125 mL) at a time. Cook mixture, stirring occasionally, until broth is almost absorbed. Continue additions of stock, cooking and stirring occasionally, until mixture becomes creamy and rice is tender. (The total cooking time should be about 20 minutes). Remove from heat. Stir in cheese, pepper and nutmeg. Taste and adjust seasonings.

NUTRITIONAL ANALYSIS	Energy	Protein	Carbohydrate	Fat	Iron
per 1/4 cup (50 mL)	38.1 kcal	1.8 g	3.5 g	1.8 g	0.17 mg

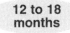

12 to 18 months

Makes 9 cups (2.25 L)

Fiesta Tomato Surprise

Kitchen Tip

This is a quick and easy meal. Use whatever kind of noodles you like.

1 lb	lean ground beef	500 g
1 lb	dried rotini or other spiral pasta	500 g
2	cans (10 oz [284 mL]) Campbell's Fiesta tomato soup	2
Half	soup can of water	Half
1 tbsp	grated Parmesan cheese	15 mL

1. In a large skillet, cook ground beef over medium-high heat until browned. Remove from heat and drain excess fat.

2. Meanwhile, in a large pot of boiling water, cook noodles according to package directions or until tender but firm. Drain. Add cooked beef, soup and water. Heat for 5 minutes or until warmed through. Serve garnished with Parmesan cheese.

NUTRITIONAL ANALYSIS	Energy	Protein	Carbohydrate	Fat	Iron
per 1/2 cup (125 mL)	171 kcal	8.5 g	23.2 g	4.7 g	1.36 mg

12 to 18 months

Serves 4

Sunshine Carrots

The "sunshine" in these carrots refers to their bright orange glaze.
Adding a pinch of sugar helps to mellows any bitterness, which makes
the humble carrot even more attractive to small children.

4	medium carrots, peeled and cut diagonally into 1-inch (2.5 cm) thick slices	4
1 tsp	granulated sugar	5 mL
1/2 tsp	cornstarch	2 mL
1/8 tsp	salt	0.5 mL
1/8 tsp	ground ginger	0.5 mL
2 tbsp	orange juice	25 mL
1 tbsp	butter *or* margarine	15 mL

1. In a saucepan cook carrots in boiling water for 10 minutes or until tender. Drain.

2. Meanwhile, in a small saucepan, combine sugar, cornstarch, salt and ginger. Add orange juice and cook, stirring constantly, until mixture thickens. Boil for 1 minute. Stir in butter, pour over carrots; toss evenly to coat.

NUTRITIONAL ANALYSIS	Energy	Protein	Carbohydrate	Fat	Iron
per serving	65 kcal	0.8 g	9.4 g	3.1 g	0.38 mg

12 to 18 months

Serves 4 adults
Makes 12 baby servings
or 3 cups (750 mL)

Ratatouille

This traditional French vegetable dish is chock -full of vitamins and minerals. It's sure to please young ones, served hot, on a cold winter night.

2 tbsp	vegetable oil	25 mL
1	clove garlic, minced	1
1/2 cup	sliced onion	125 mL
1/2 cup	diced green pepper	125 mL
2	small zucchini, peeled and sliced	2
Half	eggplant, peeled and thinly sliced	Half
2	tomatoes, peeled and diced	2
1/2 tsp	salt	2 mL
1/4 tsp	freshly ground black pepper	1 mL
Pinch	granulated sugar	Pinch

1. In a heavy-bottomed saucepan, heat oil over medium-high heat. Add garlic and the onion; sauté until softened. Add green pepper and cook until soft. Gently stir in zucchini, eggplant and tomatoes. Reduce heat to low; cover and simmer, stirring occasionally, for about 45 minutes. Serve hot or cold.

NUTRITIONAL ANALYSIS	Energy	Protein	Carbohydrate	Fat	Iron
per 1/4 cup (50 mL)	36 kcal	0.6 g	3.3 g	2.6 g	0.33 mg

12 to 18 months

Makes 4 cups (1 L)

Four-Cheese Pasta with Vegetables

Kitchen Tip

Use fontina, mozzarella and Parmesan cheeses for the kids, then add gorgonzola (or another cheese) for adult portions.

3 tbsp	butter *or* margarine	45 mL
1 1/2 tbsp	all-purpose flour	22 mL
1/4 tsp	ground nutmeg	1 mL
1/8 tsp	salt	0.5 mL
1/8 tsp	freshly ground black pepper	0.5 mL
3/4 cup	light (10 %) cream	175 mL
3/4 cup	vegetable stock	175 mL
1/3 cup	shredded fontina cheese	75 mL
1/3 cup	shredded mozzarella cheese	75 mL
1/3 cup	grated Parmesan cheese	75 mL
1/4 cup	crumbled gorgonzola or blue cheese (see Tip)	50 mL
1/2 lb	medium shell pasta or rotini	250 g
1 cup	finely chopped cooked vegetables	250 mL

1. In a saucepan melt butter over low heat. Whisk in flour, nutmeg, salt and pepper; cook for 1 minute. Whisk in cream and vegetable broth; cook, whisking constantly, for 5 minutes or until mixture is smooth and thickened. Add fontina, mozzarella and Parmesan cheeses; stir until cheese is melted.

2. Meanwhile, in a large amount of boiling water, cook pasta according to package directions until tender but firm. Drain. Add cheese sauce and cooked vegetables; toss well to combine.

3. Serve children's portions, then add gorgonzola; cover for a few minutes until gorgonzola is melted. Stir well and serve.

NUTRITIONAL ANALYSIS	Energy	Protein	Carbohydrate	Fat	Iron
per 1/2 cup (125 mL)	200 kcal	8.5 g	20.0 g	9.4 g	0.62 mg

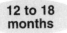

12 to 18 months

Spinach Cheese Bake

Makes 4 cups (1 L)
Serves 8

So delicious, you'll probably have to double the recipe! Be prepared to share it with others – who are bound to ask you for the recipe as soon as they taste this dish.

Kitchen Tip

You can make this dish using any number of different cheeses. If your child prefers stronger flavors, try old instead of medium Cheddar.

PREHEAT OVEN TO 350° F (180° C)

CASSEROLE

1 tbsp	butter *or* margarine	15 mL
2	eggs	2
3/4 cup	whole milk	175 mL
1/4 cup	all-purpose flour	50 mL
1/2 tsp	baking powder	2 mL
1/4 tsp	salt	1 mL
1/8 tsp	ground nutmeg	1/2 mL
1	pkg (10 oz [284 g]) fresh spinach, rough stems removed, chopped	1
2 cups	grated medium Cheddar cheese	500 mL

1. Place butter in casserole and set in oven for about 2 minutes or until it is just melted. Set aside.

2. In a large bowl, beat eggs lightly. Stir in milk. Add flour, baking powder, salt and nutmeg; beat until mixture is smooth. Stir in spinach. Add cheese. Place in prepared casserole and bake for 30 to 35 minutes.

NUTRITIONAL ANALYSIS	Energy	Protein	Carbohydrate	Fat	Iron
per 1/2 cup (125 mL)	331 kcal	20.0 g	5.9 g	25.5 g	1.87 mg

12 to 18 months

Serves 4 adults
Makes 16 baby servings

DINNER

Tuna Noodle Casserole

This soft vegetable and pasta combination is a real treat for young children.

PREHEAT OVEN TO 350° F (180° C)
CASSEROLE

1 lb	rotini or other pasta	500 g
2 tbsp	vegetable oil	25 mL
1	medium onion, chopped	1
1 or 2	cloves garlic, chopped	1 or 2
1	green pepper, diced	1
2 cups	sliced mushrooms	500 mL
2	cans (each 6.5 oz [184 g]) tuna, drained	2
2/3 cup	sliced pitted green olives (optional)	150 mL
1 1/2 cups	condensed cream of mushroom soup	375 mL
1/4 cup	grated Parmesan cheese	50 mL

1. In a large saucepan of boiling water, cook pasta according to package directions or until tender but firm.

2. In a large skillet, heat oil over medium heat. Add onions, garlic, green pepper and mushrooms; cook for 5 to 7 minutes or until vegetables begin to soften. Add tuna and sliced olives; cook for about 1 minute.

3. Transfer pasta to casserole. Add vegetable-tuna mixture and toss together. Pour soup over and top with Parmesan cheese. Bake in preheated oven for 1 hour.

NUTRITIONAL ANALYSIS	Energy	Protein	Carbohydrate	Fat	Iron
per baby serving	100 kcal	5.8 g	10.0 g	4.0 g	0.77 mg

12 to 18 months

Serves 12 adults

Makes 11 cups (2.75 L)

Baked Beans

PREHEAT OVEN TO 300° F (160° C)

DEEP BAKING DISH

Kitchen Tip

This dish is a great source of iron and protein.

If you prefer, omit the bacon.

Freeze in small portions for quick use later on.

1 1/2 lbs	dried navy beans	750 g
1/4 cup	molasses	50 mL
1/4 cup	packed brown sugar	50 mL
1	can (28 oz [796 mL]) tomatoes	1
1 tbsp	dry mustard	15 mL
1 tsp	freshly ground black pepper	5 mL
1	onion, chopped	1
1/2 tsp	salt	2 mL
8	strips bacon, chopped	8

1. In a large saucepan, soak beans in 3 times the quantity of water for 12 hours or overnight. Drain and rinse. Add fresh water to cover and bring to a boil. Reduce heat to low; cover and simmer for 1 hour. Transfer beans to baking dish.

2. Stir in molasses, brown sugar, tomatoes, mustard, pepper, onion, salt and bacon. Bake, covered, in preheated oven for 3 hours, adding water several times as needed to keep the beans moist.

NUTRITIONAL ANALYSIS	Energy	Protein	Carbohydrate	Fat	Iron
per 1/4 cup (50 mL)	78 kcal	4.4 g	13.8 g	0.9 g	1.54 mg

12 to 18 months

Serves 4 adults
Makes 16 baby servings

Sole and Spinach Casserole

Kitchen Tip

This is a delicious fish recipe that freezes well.

If you really love the flavor of fish, double the quantity called for in the recipe. The rest of the ingredients remain the same.

Fresh or frozen fish will work equally well here; just adjust the poaching time.

Poaching is a method of cooking food gently in a liquid just below the boiling point. Use enough liquid just to cover the food.

Don't be discouraged by the number of steps in this recipe – it is really very simple to prepare!

PREHEAT BROILER
CASSEROLE

14 oz	fillets of sole or other white fish	400 g
	Seasoned Spinach	
1 1/2 cups	spinach, trimmed and washed, but not dried	375 mL
1 tsp	soy sauce (low sodium)	5 mL
1 tsp	butter *or* margarine	5 mL
1/2 tsp	salt	2 mL
1/4 tsp	freshly ground black pepper	1 mL
1 tbsp	all-purpose flour	15 mL
	White Sauce	
1 tbsp	butter *or* margarine	15 mL
1 1/2 tbsp	all-purpose flour	22 mL
1 cup	whole milk	250 mL
1/2 tsp	salt	2 mL
1/2 tsp	freshly ground black pepper	2 mL
	Mushrooms	
1 tbsp	butter *or* margarine	15 mL
1 tbsp	olive oil	15 mL
2 cups	sliced mushrooms	500 mL
1/4 cup	grated Parmesan cheese	50 mL

1. In a skillet or poacher or steamer, poach sole until it flakes with a fork. (See Tip.) Drain.

2. Seasoned Spinach: In a large saucepan over high heat, cook spinach (with no more water than is clinging to the leaves) until soft. Add soy sauce, butter, salt and pepper. Sprinkle 1 tbsp (15 mL) flour over spinach and stir thoroughly to absorb any excess liquid.

3. White Sauce: In a large skillet over low heat, melt 1 tbsp (15 mL) of the butter. Stir in 1 1/2 tbsp (22 mL) of the flour; cook, stirring, for 3 to 5 minutes. Slowly whisk in milk; cook, whisking constantly, until sauce is thickened and smooth. Add salt and pepper.

4. Mushrooms: In a small skillet over medium–high heat, melt butter and olive oil. Add mushrooms and cook for about 5 minutes or until softened. Set aside.

5. Spread seasoned spinach in a layer on bottom of casserole. Arrange poached sole fillets on top of spinach. Sprinkle mushrooms over sole. Pour white sauce over. Sprinkle with Parmesan cheese. Broil until white sauce starts to bubble.

NUTRITIONAL ANALYSIS	Energy	Protein	Carbohydrate	Fat	Iron
per baby serving	65 kcal	5.6 g	2.4 g	3.7 g	0.57 mg

Serves 5 or 6
Makes 18 baby (2-inch [5 cm] square) servings

Kitchen Tip

Make sure that infant portions have noodles cut into small bites, and are allowed to cool before serving.

This version of lasagna lacks the usual cottage cheese, since it's not part of Mexican cuisine. You can add it back, if you wish: Use 1 cup (250 mL), divided between layers of noodles.

Food Safety Tip

Always use separate cutting boards for meats, poultry, fruits and vegetables, and breads. Clean cutting boards in the dishwasher or scrub with hot water and detergent after each use.

DINNER

Mexican Lasagna

Everyone knows the Italian version of lasagna. But in this recipe we add a new twist with Mexican flavors, which children particularly seem to enjoy.

PREHEAT OVEN TO 350° F (180° C)
11- BY 7-INCH (2 L) BAKING PAN, GREASED

1 tsp	vegetable oil	5 mL
1 lb	lean ground beef	500 g
1/2 cup	finely chopped onion	125 mL
1/2 cup	finely chopped green pepper	125 mL
1	can (7 1/2 oz [213 mL]) tomato sauce	1
1/2 cup	water	125 mL
1 to 2 tsp	chili powder	5 to 10 mL
1/2 tsp	salt	2 mL
1/2 tsp	dried oregano	2 mL
1/2 tsp	garlic powder	2 mL
6	cooked lasagna noodles	6
2 cups	shredded Monterey Jack cheese	500 mL

1. In a large nonstick skillet, heat oil over medium heat. Add ground beef and cook for 10 minutes or until no longer pink; drain fat. Stir in onion and green pepper; cook for 5 minutes longer or until vegetables are tender. Add tomato sauce, water, chili powder, salt, oregano and garlic powder; cook for about 10 minutes.

2. Arrange 3 noodles in bottom of prepared pan. Spoon half of sauce and half of cheese over noodles. Repeat layers.

3. Bake in preheated oven for 25 minutes or until cheese melts and casserole is bubbling. Remove from oven and let stand for 10 minutes before cutting.

NUTRITIONAL ANALYSIS	Energy	Protein	Carbohydrate	Fat	Iron
per baby serving	185 kcal	12.8 g	3.2 g	13.4 g	0.97 mg

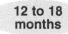

12 to 18 months

Makes 7 cups (875 mL)

Great Spaghetti Sauce

Kitchen Tip

Freeze in this sauce in batches to have on hand for a quick pasta meal.

Serve over your child's favorite pasta. Good choices include rotini or gemilli (spiral pasta).

1 tbsp	vegetable oil	15 mL
1 lb	lean ground beef	500 g
2 3/4 cups	prepared tomato sauce	675 mL
1	can (19 oz [540 mL] whole tomatoes with Italian seasoning	1
1 tbsp	granulated sugar	15 mL
1 tbsp	garlic powder	15 mL
1 tbsp	dried basil	15 mL

1. In a large skillet, heat oil over high heat. Add beef and cook until brown and cooked through. Drain fat. Reduce heat to medium. Add tomato sauce, tomatoes, sugar, garlic powder and basil; cook, uncovered, for 10 to 15 minutes.

NUTRITIONAL ANALYSIS per 1/4 cup (50 mL)	Energy	Protein	Carbohydrate	Fat	Iron
	78 kcal	7.1 g	56 g	4.4 g	0.71 mg

Makes about 22 meatballs

DINNER

Meatballs and Mushrooms

Kitchen Tip

This dish is a good source of iron. It also freezes well.

Serve over pasta, such as linguine (cut up for children), or with rice.

Soft meat in a nicely herbed sauce make this a child's favorite.

2 tsp	vegetable oil or olive oil	10 mL
2 cups	sliced mushrooms	500 mL
2 tsp	chopped fresh dill or basil (or 1 tsp [5 mL] dried)	10 mL
1/4 tsp	salt	1 mL
1/4 tsp	freshly ground black pepper	1 mL
2/3 cup	evaporated milk, divided	150 mL
1/4 cup	cornflake crumbs	50 mL
1/4 cup	finely chopped onion	50 mL
1/4 tsp	ground allspice	1 mL
1/4 tsp	ground nutmeg	1 mL
19 oz	lean ground beef	575 g
4 tsp	all-purpose flour	20 mL
2/3 cup	beef stock	150 mL

1. In a large skillet, heat oil over medium-high heat. Add mushrooms, dill and a pinch of the salt and pepper; sauté for 8 to 10 minutes or until brown. Transfer to a bowl and set aside.

2. In another bowl, combine 2 tbsp (25 mL) of the milk with cereal crumbs, onion, allspice, nutmeg and the remaining salt and pepper. Add beef; mix well. With your hands, shape into meatballs, about 1 inch (2.5 cm) in diameter.

3. Return skillet to heat and add meatballs; cook for 8 to 10 minutes or until they are brown. Add reserved mushrooms. Stir in flour. Add stock and remaining milk. Bring to a boil. Simmer, stirring, for another 5 minutes or until thickened.

NUTRITIONAL ANALYSIS	Energy	Protein	Carbohydrate	Fat	Iron
per meatball	75 kcal	5.7 g	1.8 g	5.0 g	0.69 mg

Serves 8 adults

Makes 20 baby servings

Easy Meatballs

Here's a recipe that kids love. Serve over rice or pasta, or serve with bread that children can use for dipping.

Kitchen Tip

This recipe is a great source of iron. It freezes well, too.

2 lbs	ground beef	1 kg
2	eggs	2
1/2 tsp	salt	2 mL
1/2 tsp	freshly ground black pepper	2 mL
1/2 cup	water	125 mL
1/2 cup	bread crumbs	125 mL
1 tbsp	lemon juice	15 mL
1/2 cup	granulated sugar	125 mL
2 cups	water	500 mL
2 1/2 cups	tomato juice	625 mL
3	celery stalks, diced	3
1	small onion, diced	1
1	can (2.8 oz [80 mL]) tomato paste	1

1. In a large bowl, combine ground beef, eggs, salt, pepper, 1/2 cup (125 mL) water and bread crumbs. Mix well. With your hands, roll meat mixture into 1-inch (2.5 cm) meatballs. Set aside.

2. In a large saucepan over medium-high heat, combine lemon juice, sugar, 2 cups (500 mL) water, tomato juice, celery and onion; cook, covered, for 30 minutes. Reduce heat to simmer. Add meatballs and tomato paste; cook, uncovered, for 2 hours.

NUTRITIONAL ANALYSIS	Energy	Protein	Carbohydrate	Fat	Iron
per baby serving	181 kcal	10.2 g	7.9 g	11.1 g	1.4 mg

12 to 18 months

Makes 3 cups (750 mL)

Cheese Tortellini with Mixed Vegetables

Tortellini is probably the most child-friendly of pastas – easy for little fingers to pick up without the need for a fork or spoon. Messy, but fun!

1 cup	tomato sauce	250 mL
1	small clove garlic, minced (optional)	1
1/2 tsp	dried basil	2 mL
1/2 tsp	dried oregano	2 mL
1/8 tsp	granulated sugar	0.5 mL
1/8 tsp	salt	0.5
1/8 tsp	freshly ground black pepper	0.5
2 cups	frozen cheese tortellini	500 mL
1 cup	frozen mixed vegetables	250 mL
2 tbsp	grated Parmesan cheese	25 mL

1. In a saucepan combine tomato sauce, garlic (if using), basil, oregano, sugar, salt and pepper. Bring to a boil. Reduce heat to low and simmer, covered and stirring occasionally, for 10 minutes.

2. Meanwhile, bring a large saucepan of water to a boil. Add tortellini, return to a boil and cook according to package directions. During the last 5 minutes of cooking, add mixed vegetables; continue to cook until vegetables are tender. Drain well.

3. Toss drained tortellini with tomato sauce and serve sprinkled with cheese.

NUTRITIONAL ANALYSIS	Energy	Protein	Carbohydrate	Fat	Iron
per 1/2 cup (125 mL)	157 kcal	8.9 g	19.3 g	5.4 g	1.00 mg

12 to 18 months

Serves 4 adults
Makes 12 baby servings

Crustless Tofu Quiche

Tofu takes on the flavors of its accompanying vegetables
in this crustless quiche.

Kitchen Tip

The optional tomato provides
added color to this dish.

Firm tofu will also work in this
recipe, but the silken variety will
give it a smoother texture.

PREHEAT OVEN TO 350° F (180° C)
8-INCH (20 CM) PIE PLATE, GREASED

2	eggs	2
1 cup	cubed drained silken tofu	250 mL
1 tbsp	all-purpose flour	15 mL
2 tsp	lemon juice *or* 2% milk	10 mL
1/8 tsp	ground nutmeg	0.5 mL
1/8 tsp	salt	0.5 mL
1/8 tsp	freshly ground black pepper	0.5 mL
1/2 cup	finely chopped frozen mixed vegetables, thawed	125 mL
1 tbsp	butter or margarine, melted	15 mL
1/2 cup	fresh whole wheat bread crumbs	125 mL
2 tbsp	grated Parmesan cheese	25 mL
1	medium tomato (optional), cut into wedges	1

1. In a food processor or blender, combine eggs and tofu; process until smooth. Add flour, juice and seasonings; blend to combine. Transfer to bowl; stir in chopped vegetables.

2. In a bowl combine melted butter and bread crumbs. Press into bottom of prepared pan. Pour tofu mixture over bread crumbs. Sprinkle with cheese. Bake in preheated oven for 35 minutes or until set in center. Arrange tomato wedges, if using, around outer edge; bake for 5 minutes longer to warm tomatoes.

3. Cut quiche into 4 wedges for adults, 12 for babies.

NUTRITIONAL ANALYSIS	Energy	Protein	Carbohydrate	Fat	Iron
per baby serving	68 kcal	4.0 g	5.7 g	3.4 g	1.67 mg

12 to 18 months

Serves 4 adults
Makes 12 baby servings

Cheese and Vegetable Quiche

Kitchen Tip

If you prefer, make this quiche in a square baking pan; cut into small squares to serve as appetizers.

Quiche is so delicious and versatile, it should be part of every family cook's repertoire. This one is particularly healthy, with the traditional pastry replaced by a bread crumb crust. Any small pieces left after dinner can be used as a snack. It is a good way to add cottage cheese to a child's diet.

PREHEAT OVEN TO 350° F (180° C)
9-INCH [23 CM] PIE PLATE, GREASED

1	slice whole wheat bread	1
2 tbsp	melted butter or margarine, divided	25 mL
1 cup	chopped spinach	250 mL
1 cup	chopped mushrooms	250 mL
Half	red bell pepper, chopped	Half
1/2 tsp	dried basil	2 mL
1/2 tsp	dried oregano	2 mL
1/4 tsp	salt	1 mL
1/4 tsp	freshly ground black pepper	1 mL
1 cup	cottage cheese	250 mL
4	eggs, beaten	4
2/3 cup	2% milk	150 mL
1/4 cup	shredded Cheddar cheese	50 mL

1. Crumble bread into fine crumbs; toss with 1 tbsp (15 mL) of the melted butter. Sprinkle bread crumbs into prepared pan.

2. In a large skillet, melt remaining butter over medium-high heat. Add spinach, mushrooms and red pepper; cook, stirring occasionally, for 10 minutes or until vegetables are softened. Add basil, oregano, salt and pepper. Stir in cottage cheese. Spoon into pie pan.

3. In a small bowl, whisk together eggs, milk and cheese. Pour over vegetable mixture. Bake in preheated oven for 45 minutes or until puffy and set in center. Let stand for 10 minutes before cutting.

NUTRITIONAL ANALYSIS	Energy	Protein	Carbohydrate	Fat	Iron
per baby serving	82 kcal	6.2 g	3.3 g	4.9 g	0.78 mg

12 to 18 months

Serves 4

Baked Mediterranean Salmon Fillets

Adding Mediterranean flavors to succulent salmon gives a delightful twist to this favorite fish. Baking the salmon in broth ensures that the fish remains moist – which makes it easier (and more enjoyable) for children to eat.

PREHEAT OVEN TO 400° F (200° C)

8-INCH (2 L) SQUARE BAKING PAN, GREASED

1 lb	salmon fillets	500 g
1/4 tsp	dried oregano	1 mL
1/4 tsp	dried thyme	1 mL
Half	lemon, thinly sliced	Half
1	large tomato, sliced	1
Half	green pepper, diced	Half
1/4 cup	finely chopped onion	50 mL
1/2 cup	chicken stock	125 mL
1 tbsp	lemon juice	15 mL

Chopped fresh parsley (optional)

1. Arrange fish fillets in prepared baking pan. Sprinkle with oregano and thyme. Place lemon and tomato slices, green pepper and onion over fish.

2. In a small bowl, combine chicken stock and lemon juice; pour over vegetables and fish. Cover and bake in preheated oven for 20 minutes or until fish flakes easily with a fork at its thickest part. If desired, garnish with parsley before serving.

NUTRITIONAL ANALYSIS	Energy	Protein	Carbohydrate	Fat	Iron
per serving	248 kcal	35.0 g	3.8 g	9.6 g	2.04 mg

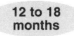
12 to 18 months

Makes 16 cakes

Simple Salmon Cakes

PREHEAT OVEN TO 375° F (190° C)
BAKING SHEET, WELL GREASED

Kitchen Tip

Try the salmon and potato mixture on its own – it's tasty and particularly appealing to younger children who still like their food a little mushy. Makes great use of leftover mashed potatoes.

2	cans (each 7 1/2 oz (213 g) salmon, bones and skin removed, drained and flaked	2
1 1/2 cups	mashed potato (about 3 medium)	375 mL
2	eggs, separated	2
2 tbsp	all-purpose flour	25 mL
Pinch	salt	Pinch
1/2 cup	dried bread crumbs	125 mL

1. In a bowl combine salmon and potato. Blend in egg yolks. With your hands, form mixture into flat cakes. Dust each cake with a mixture of flour and salt. Brush cakes with egg white. Coat with bread crumbs and bake in preheated oven for 15 minutes or until golden brown.

NUTRITIONAL ANALYSIS	Energy	Protein	Carbohydrate	Fat	Iron
per cake	80 kcal	7.1 g	6.2 g	2.8 g	0.57 mg

12 to 18 months

Serves 4 adults
Makes 10 baby servings

DINNER

Fish, Tomato and Spinach Casserole

Kitchen Tip

Beloved even by finicky eaters, this recipe can be prepared in advance and cooked before serving.

PREHEAT OVEN TO 350° F (180° C)

CASSEROLE

1	pkg (10 oz [284 g] fresh spinach, washed, coarse stems removed	1
2 cups	tomato sauce	500 mL
13 oz	frozen cod or sole, thawed	400 g
2 cups	grated mozzarella or white Cheddar cheese	500 mL

1. In a saucepan over medium-high heat, cook wet spinach leaves for 5 to 8 minutes until just limp. Drain, squeeze out remaining moisture and chop coarsely.

2. Pour half of tomato sauce into casserole. Create layers of fish, then spinach, then cheese, using half of each of these ingredients. Repeat layers with remainder of ingredients, starting with tomato sauce and ending with cheese.

3. Bake in preheated oven for 45 minutes or until bubbling.

NUTRITIONAL ANALYSIS	Energy	Protein	Carbohydrate	Fat	Iron
per baby serving	195 kcal	22.0 g	6.3 g	9.2 g	1.49 mg

Serves 4 adults

Makes 12 baby slices

Cheeseburger Pie

PREHEAT OVEN TO 350° F (180° C)

9-INCH (23 CM) PIE PLATE

8 oz	lean ground beef	250 g
1/2 cup	mayonnaise	125 mL
1/2 cup	2% milk	125 mL
2	eggs, beaten	2
1 tbsp	cornstarch	15 mL
1 cup	grated Cheddar cheese	250 mL
1/3 cup	chopped green onions	75 mL
Pinch	freshly ground black pepper	Pinch
1	double pie shell, unbaked	1

1. In a skillet over medium–high heat, brown ground beef. Drain excess fat.

2. In a large bowl, combine mayonnaise, milk, eggs and cornstarch. Stir in cheese, green onions, pepper and cooked beef. Pour mixture into pie shell; cover with top crust and crimp edges. Bake in preheated oven for 40 to 50 minutes or until a knife inserted in the center comes out clean.

NUTRITIONAL ANALYSIS	Energy	Protein	Carbohydrate	Fat	Iron
per baby slice	331 kcal	9.2 g	14.7 g	26.0 g	1.30 mg

DINNER

Shepherd's Pie

Here's a soft-textured one-dish meal that your family will love

PREHEAT OVEN TO 375° F (190° C)

9- BY 13-INCH (3 L) BAKING DISH

1 tsp	vegetable oil	5 mL
1 1/2 lbs	lean ground beef	750 g
2 tbsp	chopped onion	25 mL
1/4 tsp	salt	1 mL
1/4 tsp	mixed dried herbs (parsley, thyme, sage)	1 mL
1 1/4 cups	gravy *or* bouillon	300 mL
1	can (12 oz [341 mL]) corn kernels	1
2 cups	mashed potatoes	500 mL
1/4 cup	grated Cheddar cheese	50 mL

1. In a large skillet, heat oil over medium–high heat. Add beef and cook until browned. Add onion and cook for 3 minutes or until softened. Stir in salt, herbs, gravy and corn.

2. Pour beef mixture into baking dish and cover with mashed potatoes. Bake in preheated oven for 30 to 35 minutes or until potatoes are browned. Top with cheese and bake for another 5 minutes.

NUTRITIONAL ANALYSIS	Energy	Protein	Carbohydrate	Fat	Iron
per baby serving	102 kcal	0.1 g	5.9 g	5.6 g	0.82 mg

Easy Meatloaf

PREHEAT OVEN TO 350° F (180° C)
9- BY 5-INCH (2 L) LOAF PAN, GREASED

Kitchen Tip

The ketchup topping makes a
tangy crust that your children
will love.

1 lb	ground beef	500 g
1	egg	1
	Salt and freshly ground black pepper to taste	
Half	onion, chopped	Half
1/4 cup	bread crumbs	50 mL
1/4 cup	ketchup	50 mL
1 tsp	HP sauce	5 mL
	Additional ketchup for topping	

1. In a large bowl, combine beef, egg, salt and pepper, onion, bread crumbs, 1/4 cup (50 mL) ketchup and HP sauce. Mix well and transfer to prepared loaf pan. Cover top with additional ketchup. Bake for 1 hour or until juices run clear.

NUTRITIONAL ANALYSIS	Energy	Protein	Carbohydrate	Fat	Iron
per 1 slice	129 kcal	8.2 g	2.7 g	9.2 g	0.96 mg

12 to 18 months

Serves 4 adults
Makes 12 baby servings

DINNER

Chicken Pot Pie

This old-fashioned meal will be a big winner,
especially on cold winter nights.

PREHEAT OVEN TO 400° F (200° C)

2 tbsp	butter *or* margarine	25 mL
1/3 cup	all-purpose flour	75 mL
1 1/2 cups	chicken stock	375 mL
1 1/2 cups	2 % milk	375 mL
2 cups	cubed cooked chicken	500 mL
1 cup	diced cooked turnips	250 mL
1 cup	diced cooked carrots	250 mL
1 cup	frozen peas, thawed	250 mL
1/4 tsp	dried thyme	2 mL
Dash	cayenne pepper	Dash
1/4 tsp	freshly ground black pepper	2 mL
1 tsp	salt (omit if using canned chicken broth or bouillon)	5 mL
1	double pie shell (unbaked)	1

1. In a large saucepan, melt butter over medium heat. Whisk in flour, stock and milk. Bring to a boil, whisking constantly. Reduce heat to low and simmer for 5 minutes or until smooth and thickened. Stir in chicken, turnips, carrots, peas, thyme, cayenne pepper, black pepper and salt.

2. Pour mixture into unbaked pie shell. Cover with pastry top and crimp the edges. Cut steam holes in the top. Bake in preheated oven for 20 minutes; reduce heat to 350° F (180° C) and bake for another 40 minutes or until pastry is browned.

NUTRITIONAL ANALYSIS	Energy	Protein	Carbohydrate	Fat	Iron
per baby slice	261 kcal	12.2 g	22.0 g	13.7 g	1.53 mg

Serves 8

Chicken Thighs with Herbs

Kitchen Tip

This dish is a very good source of iron. Young children enjoy it because the thighs are soft and never dry.

PREHEAT OVEN TO 375° F (190° C)

CASSEROLE OR BAKING DISH, GREASED

3 tbsp	mayonnaise	45 mL
2 tbsp	Dijon mustard	25 mL
1 tbsp	lemon juice	15 mL
1 tsp	dried rosemary, crushed	5 mL
1 tsp	dried basil	5 mL
1 tsp	dried thyme	5 mL
1 tsp	dried savory	5 mL
2 tsp	grated Parmesan cheese	10 mL
2 cups	crushed cornflake-type cereal	500 mL
1/4 tsp	freshly ground black pepper	1 mL
8	boneless skinless chicken thighs	8

1. In a small bowl, combine mayonnaise, mustard, lemon juice, herbs and Parmesan cheese.

2. In a medium bowl, mix cornflakes with pepper.

3. Dip chicken thighs one at a time into the mayonnaise/herb mixture, then into cereal mixture, making sure each is well coated. Place thighs in prepared baking dish and bake for 35 to 40 minutes or until juices run clear when pierced with a fork.

NUTRITIONAL ANALYSIS	Energy	Protein	Carbohydrate	Fat	Iron
per serving	150 kcal	14.6 g	6.2 g	7.2 g	2.03 mg

over 18 months

Makes about 4 cups (1 L)

Kitchen Tip

For a change of flavor, use Dijon or dried mustard.

Chickpea and Red Pepper Salad

This salad offers a delicious mix of flavors that surprises everyone – even those that don't usually eat chickpeas!

2	cans (each 19 oz [540 mL]) chickpeas, rinsed and drained	2
2	red bell peppers, finely chopped	2
3	green onions, chopped	3
	Dressing	
2 tbsp	balsamic vinegar	25 mL
2 tbsp	vegetable oil	25 mL
2 tsp	prepared mustard	10 mL
1 tsp	dried basil	5 mL

1. In a bowl combine chickpeas with red peppers and green onions.

2. Dressing: In a small bowl, whisk together vinegar, oil, mustard and basil. Drizzle over salad and toss.

NUTRITIONAL ANALYSIS	Energy	Protein	Carbohydrate	Fat	Iron
per 1/4 cup (50 mL)	92 kcal	4.4 g	13.5 g	2.5 g	1.43 mg

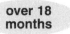

Makes 1 cup (250 mL)

Honey Salad Dressing

Kids will love this tangy dressing. It can be used on salads,
as a vegetable dip, or as a dipping sauce for baked fish or fish sticks.

3/4 cup	mayonnaise	175 mL
1 1/2 tbsp	red wine vinegar	22 mL
1 1/2 tbsp	liquid honey	22 mL
1	clove garlic, crushed	1
2 tsp	Dijon mustard	10 mL
1 tsp	Worcestershire sauce	5 mL
1/4 tsp	Tabasco sauce	1 mL
1/4 tsp	salt	1 mL
1/4 tsp	freshly ground black pepper	1 mL

1. In a bowl whisk together all ingredients until thoroughly blended. Use to dress salad or as a dip for vegetables.

NUTRITIONAL ANALYSIS	Energy	Protein	Carbohydrate	Fat	Iron
per 1 tablespoon (15 mL)	82 kcal	0.2 g	1.9 g	17.2 g	0.14 mg

over 18 months

Makes 4 1/2 cups (1.125 L)

DINNER

Rice Salad

This tasty, sweet rice salad is a great accompaniment to just about any meat or fish.

Variations

Replace half the diced celery with diced red or green pepper.

Add 1 tsp (5mL) curry powder to the dressing for a different taste

3 cups	cooked white rice	750 mL
1/2 cup	diced celery	125 mL
1/2 cup	chopped onion	125 mL
10 oz	peas (canned or frozen), drained	300 g
1/4 cup	vegetable oil	50 mL
2 tbsp	granulated sugar	25 mL
2 tbsp	low-sodium soy sauce	25 mL
1 1/2 tbsp	rice vinegar	22 mL

1. In a large bowl, combine rice, celery, onion and peas.
2. In a small bowl, whisk together oil, sugar, soy sauce and vinegar. Pour dressing over rice. Toss and let stand for at least 1 hour before serving.

NUTRITIONAL ANALYSIS	Energy	Protein	Carbohydrate	Fat	Iron
per 1/4 cup (50 mL)	69 kcal	1.5 g	10.4 g	2.4 g	0.34 mg

Chicken and Peach Salad

Serving Tip

Children will probably love the peach and chicken mixture, but certainly try them on some romaine lettuce as well.

Food Safety Tip

Always check the label for the "best before " date or the "packaged on" date when purchasing chicken. When you get home, immediately freeze any chicken you do not intend to use within 1 to 3 days. Enclose the packages in plastic freezer bags or over-wrap them with heavy-duty foil.

Maximum storage times for chicken in the refrigerator (40° F [4° C]): 1 day for ground chicken; 2 to 3 days for whole chicken or chicken pieces; and 3 to 4 days for cooked chicken.

Maximum storage times for chicken in the freezer (0° F [-18° C]): 2 to 3 months for ground chicken; 6 months for chicken pieces; 12 months for a whole chicken; and 2 to 3 months for cooked chicken.

Serve this tasty salad when peaches are in season and at their best. A whole wheat roll or toast finishes the meal.

2	cooked chicken breasts (half breasts), cut into slivers	2
2	ripe peaches, peeled and sliced	2
2	green onions, sliced	2
2 tbsp	orange juice	25 mL
2 tbsp	mayonnaise	25 mL
1 tbsp	red wine vinegar	15 mL
	Romaine lettuce	
1 to 2 tbsp	chopped fresh basil leaves (optional)	15 to 25 mL

1. In a bowl combine chicken, peaches and green onions.

2. In a small container with a tight-fitting lid, shake together juice, mayonnaise and vinegar. Pour dressing over chicken mixture; toss lightly to coat. Cover and refrigerate for 30 minutes or longer.

3. Tear lettuce into small pieces and arrange in a serving bowl. Top with chicken mixture; sprinkle with basil, if using, and serve.

NUTRITIONAL ANALYSIS	Energy	Protein	Carbohydrate	Fat	Iron
per serving	186 kcal	18.9 g	8.8 g	8.3 g	1.25 mg

over 18 months

Makes 6 cups (1.5 L)

Pasta Primavera

Kitchen Tip

Fusilli and rotini worked well for this dish, but any kind of pasta will do.

3 cups	fusilli *or* rotini	750 mL
3 1/2 cups	mixed vegetables (fresh or frozen, thawed)	875 mL
1	can (12 oz [385 mL]) evaporated milk	1
1 cup	shredded old Cheddar cheese	250 mL
1/2 cup	grated Parmesan cheese	125 mL
4	slices ham, cut into thin strips	4
	Salt and freshly ground black pepperto taste	

1. In a large pot of boiling water, cook pasta according to package directions or until tender but firm. Add vegetables and cook for 5 minutes. Drain. Return pasta and vegetables to the pot.

2. Over medium high heat, gently add the evaporated milk, Cheddar cheese, Parmesan cheese and ham. Cook, stirring, until cheese has melted and sauce thickens. Season to taste with salt and pepper.

NUTRITIONAL ANALYSIS per 1/2 cup (125 mL)	Energy	Protein	Carbohydrate	Fat	Iron
	177 kcal	10.9 g	19.5 g	6.3 g	0.89 mg

over 18 months

Serves 3

Oven-Roasted Potato Wedges

Kitchen Tip

Packaged herb blends can be found in the seasonings section of most supermarkets. Or make your own.

These roast potato wedges are as crisp as French fries. They're just right for dipping into things like ketchup, salsa or a creamy Red Pepper Dip (see recipe, page 228). They are also excellent served on their own as an accompaniment to a dinner entrée. Try the same thing with carrots, zucchini or sweet potatoes.

NONSTICK BAKING SHEET

PREHEAT OVEN TO 400° F (200° C)

1 lb	baking potatoes, scrubbed and cut into wedges	500 g
2 tbsp	vegetable oil	25 mL
1 tbsp	garlic and herb blend (see Tip)	15 mL

1. In a large bowl, toss potatoes with oil and seasonings. Spread in a single layer on a baking sheet. Bake in oven for 40 minutes, turning halfway through cooking time, until potatoes are crisp on the outside and tender on the inside.

NUTRITIONAL ANALYSIS	Energy	Protein	Carbohydrate	Fat	Iron
per serving	232 kcal	3.7 g	38.0 g	7.9 g	0.66 mg

over 18 months

Makes 3 1/2 cups (875 mL)

Zucchini and Feta Sauté

Kitchen Tips

If feta is too strong for your child, you may want to try a milder cheese, such as Cheddar.

Serve this dish with bread. It's also delicious over pasta.

1/4 cup	butter *or* margarine	50 mL
1/2 cup	chopped onions	125 mL
1/2 tsp	salt	2 mL
1/2 tsp	dried basil	2 mL
1/8 tsp	garlic powder	0.5 mL
3 cups	shredded unpeeled zucchini	750 mL
1 cup	diced tomatoes	250 mL
1 cup	crumbled feta cheese	250 mL
1/4 cup	Parmesan cheese	50 mL

1. In a large skillet, melt the butter over medium heat. Stir in onions, salt, basil and garlic powder; cook, uncovered, for 5 minutes or until onions are soft. Add zucchini and cook, stirring occasionally, for 2 to 3 minutes.

2. Sprinkle tomatoes and cheese over the zucchini. Cover and cook for another 2 minutes.

NUTRITIONAL ANALYSIS	Energy	Protein	Carbohydrate	Fat	Iron
per 1/2 cup (125 mL)	184 kcal	7.4 g	7.0 g	14.6 g	0.78 mg

over 18 months

Serves 4 adults

Makes 16 baby servings

Chicken and Vegetables

This as an absolute must-try recipe. It is incredibly quick and easy to make. Your whole family will enjoy this and tastes great the next day.

Kitchen Tip

Add other vegetables – such as sliced zucchini or green or red bell peppers – for additional flavor and color.

PREHEAT OVEN TO 400° F (200° C)

CASSEROLE, GREASED

1 lb	carrots, peeled and sliced	500 g
2	sweet potatoes, sliced	2
3/4 cup	chicken stock	175 mL
1/2 tsp	salt	2 mL
1/2 tsp	freshly ground black pepper	2 mL
4	boneless skinless chicken breasts	4
4 tbsp	Dijon mustard	60 mL
1/2 tsp	dried thyme	2 mL

1. Place carrots on bottom of casserole. Arrange potatoes on top of carrots. Pour half of the stock over vegetables. Cover with foil and bake in preheated oven for 20 minutes.

2. Reduce heat to 375° F (190° C). Stir vegetables and nestle chicken among vegetables. Add salt and pepper to remaining stock. Add mustard and thyme. Pour over chicken mixture and bake for 45 minutes until chicken is no longer pink inside.

NUTRITIONAL ANALYSIS	Energy	Protein	Carbohydrate	Fat	Iron
per baby serving	68 kcal	7.8 g	7.5 g	0.7 g	0.63 mg

over 18 months

Serves 2 or 3

Asian Barbecued Tofu Cubes

Kitchen Tips

Use more or less garlic, according to taste.

If using wooden skewers, remember to soak them in water for at least 30 minutes before use. This will prevent the wood from burning on the grill.

Remove skewers before serving; they are unsafe for children under the age of 4 years.

If you substitute chicken for tofu, boil the marinade for 5 minutes before using it to brush on chicken while it is being grilled. Or discard marinade if not using.

Tofu's bland taste gives it the ability to take on the flavor of foods with which it is cooked. In this recipe, tofu cubes adopt the Asian tastes of its marinade – soy, garlic and ginger root. While tofu is a mainstay of vegetarian diets, non-vegetarians will find it surprisingly tasty when prepared in this manner. However, if you still find tofu just a little too earnest, replace it with cubes of chicken. Beginning self-feeders find the cubes easy to eat.

PREHEAT GRILL TO MEDIUM

8 oz	firm tofu, cubed	250 g
1 to 2 tbsp	soy sauce (low sodium)	15 to 25 mL
Half	small garlic clove, crushed (see Tip)	Half
1 tsp	minced ginger root	5 mL
1 tsp	lemon juice	5 mL
1 tsp	olive oil	5 mL
	Metal or wooden skewers (see Tip)	

1. Place tofu cubes in a small, sealable plastic bag.

2. In a small bowl, combine soy sauce, garlic, ginger root, lemon juice and oil. Pour over tofu, seal bag and refrigerate for several hours.

3. Remove cubes from marinade and thread on skewers. Reserve marinade (you may need to boil it; see Tip). Grill skewers on preheated barbecue for 10 minutes or until crisp. Baste frequently with reserved marinade.

NUTRITIONAL ANALYSIS	Energy	Protein	Carbohydrate	Fat	Iron
per serving (of 3 total)	141 kcal	13.9 g	4.6 g	8.8 g	8.96 mg

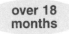

over 18 months

Serves 8

Vegetable Pizza

Kitchen Tips

Feel free to substitute carrots with other vegetables, such as blanched broccoli florets, diced zucchini, sliced mushrooms, chopped green or yellow bell peppers.

Jars of roasted red peppers are available in supermarkets. They will keep for months in the refrigerator.

This pizza starts with a store-bought shell. Add an interesting herb-cheese mixture, scatter vegetables and more cheese on top and into the oven. Deliciously easy!

PREHEAT OVEN TO 450° F (230° C)

1 tbsp	olive oil	15 mL
1 1/2 cups	shredded carrots (see Tip)	375 mL
1/4 cup	chopped fresh parsley	50 mL
2	cloves garlic, minced	2
2 tbsp	red wine vinegar or balsamic vinegar	25 mL
1 tsp	dried oregano	5 mL
1/2 tsp	dried basil	2 mL
3 cups	shredded mozzarella cheese, divided	750 mL
1	12-inch (30 cm) pizza shell	1
2 tbsp	diced roasted red pepper (see Tip)	25 mL

1. In skillet heat oil over medium heat. Add carrots and stir to coat. Sprinkle with 2 tbsp (25 mL) water; cover and cook for 5 minutes. Set aside.

2. Meanwhile, combine parsley, garlic, vinegar, oregano and basil. Combine with 2 cups (500 mL) of the cheese. Place crust on baking sheet. Spread with herb-cheese mixture. Scatter carrots and red pepper over. Top with remaining cheese. Bake in preheated oven for 15 minutes or until golden brown and cheese is melted.

NUTRITIONAL ANALYSIS	Energy	Protein	Carbohydrate	Fat	Iron
per serving	399 kcal	31.0 g	22.1 g	20.0 g	0.54 mg

over 18 months

Serves 4

Makes 4 cups (1 L)

DINNER

Creamy Fettuccine Mushroom Alfredo

Kitchen Tip

Clean mushrooms just before using. Never immerse mushrooms in water; they'll absorb the water and become mushy. It's best just to wipe with a damp paper towel. Trim a small amount from stem ends and you're ready to go.

Our version of this classic pasta dish is very quick and easy to prepare. Almost a meal in itself, you only need to add a salad or cooked vegetable!

3 tbsp	olive oil	45 mL
2 cups	sliced mushrooms (see Tip)	500 mL
1	clove garlic, minced	1
1/2 cup	light (10%) cream	125 mL
Half	pkg (8 oz [250 g]) cream cheese, cubed	Half
1/2 tsp	dried tarragon	2 mL
1/2 tsp	dried thyme	2 mL
8 oz	fettuccine	250 g
	Grated Parmesan cheese	

1. In a large skillet, heat oil over medium-high heat. Add mushrooms and garlic; sauté, stirring constantly, for 5 minutes. Reduce heat. Add cream, cream cheese, tarragon and thyme; stir until smooth and cheese has melted.

2. Meanwhile, in a large saucepan, cook fettuccine in boiling water according to package directions. Drain well and return to saucepan. Stir in mushroom sauce. Sprinkle generously with cheese.

NUTRITIONAL ANALYSIS	Energy	Protein	Carbohydrate	Fat	Iron
per 1/2 cup (125 mL)	159 kcal	3.2 g	9.4 g	12.4 g	0.75 mg

over 18 months

Makes 3 1/2 cups (875 mL)

Vegetarian Chili

Kitchen Tip

Leftover chickpeas can be used to make Hummus (see recipe, page 229).

Use red lentils in this recipe. They cook down to a nice mushy consistency that's ideal for chili.

Add chili powder after you have removed the children's portion.

Children enjoy this "good for you" vegetarian chili for the simple reason that it tastes great. So will their parents. Served with cooked brown or white rice or toast, it is a complete protein meal.

1 cup	tomato juice	250 mL
1 cup	vegetable stock *or* beef stock	250 mL
1 cup	chickpeas, drained and rinsed	250 mL
1	medium potato, diced	1
1/4 cup	dried red lentils, washed (see Tip)	50 mL
1	medium carrot, chopped	1
Half	small onion, chopped	Half
1/2 cup	finely chopped green pepper	125 mL
1	clove garlic, minced	1
1 tbsp	chili powder (see Tip)	15 mL
1/4 tsp	salt	1 mL
1/4 tsp	freshly ground black pepper	1 mL

1. In a saucepan combine tomato juice, stock, chickpeas, potato, lentils, carrot, onion, green pepper and garlic. Cover and bring to a boil. Reduce heat and simmer, covered, for about 20 minutes or until vegetables and lentils are tender. Stir frequently, since the mixture has a tendency to stick as it thickens.

2. Taste and adjust flavor by adding chili powder, salt and pepper; cook for another 5 minutes and serve.

NUTRITIONAL ANALYSIS	Energy	Protein	Carbohydrate	Fat	Iron
per 1/2 cup (125 mL)	167 kcal	8.7 g	29.8 g	2.3 g	3.03 mg

over 18 months

Serves 4

DINNER

Speedy Skillet Supper

The perfect recipe for when you have only 10 minutes to prepare dinner. Eggs, one of "nature's true convenience foods", are a principal ingredient. It also tastes good, appeals to children and is nutritious.

2 tbsp	butter *or* margarine	25 mL
1/2 cup	finely chopped onion	125 mL
1/2 cup	finely chopped green or red bell pepper	125 mL
5	eggs	5
3 tbsp	2% milk	45 mL
1/2 tsp	dried basil	2 mL
1/2 tsp	salt	2 mL
Half	pkg (8 oz [250 g]) cream cheese, cubed	Half
1	medium tomato, chopped	1
1/2 cup	diced cooked ham	125 mL
	Whole wheat toast	

1. In a skillet melt butter over medium-high heat. Add onion and green pepper; sauté for 5 minutes or until tender. Reduce heat to medium-low.

2. Meanwhile, in a small bowl, whisk together eggs, milk and seasonings. Stir in cheese and tomato.

3. Pour egg mixture and ham into skillet; cook over low heat, stirring occasionally, for 5 minutes or until eggs are cooked but still moist. Serve over toast.

NUTRITIONAL ANALYSIS	Energy	Protein	Carbohydrate	Fat	Iron
per serving	307 kcal	14.3 g	6.4 g	25.1 g	2.4 mg

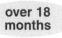

over 18 months

Makes 48

Square Chicken Meatballs

Kitchen Tips

Ground beef can replace chicken.

Freeze any leftover squares in the pan. Place pan in a plastic freezer bag for longer storage. At serving time, reheat in a microwave oven.

To make soft bread crumbs, pull fresh bread into small pieces. One slice should be sufficient for this recipe.

Food Safety Tip

When defrosting ground meats or poultry in the microwave oven, remove outside portions as they thaw. This keeps the outside from starting to cook before the inside thaws. Any meats or poultry defrosted in the microwave should be cooked immediately.

If you will not be using ground meat or poultry within 1 day, freeze it.

This recipe eliminates all the time normally required to form round meatballs. Here we simply pat the ground chicken into a pan and cut it into squares after cooking. Squares can be cut to child or adult sizes.

PREHEAT OVEN TO 400° F (200° C)

8-INCH (2 L) SQUARE BAKING PAN, GREASED

1 lb	lean ground chicken (see Tip)	500 g
1 cup	finely chopped mushrooms	250 mL
2 tbsp	finely chopped onion	25 mL
3/4 cup	soft bread crumbs (see Tip)	175 mL
1/2 tsp	dried basil	2 mL
1/2 tsp	dried thyme	2 mL
1/8 tsp	salt	0.5 mL
1/8 tsp	freshly ground black pepper	0.5 mL

1. In a bowl combine chicken, mushrooms, onion, bread crumbs, basil, thyme, salt and pepper. Pat mixture into prepared pan. Mark into small squares.

2. Bake in preheated oven for 20 minutes or until chicken is well done and juices run clear. Remove and cut into squares.

NUTRITIONAL ANALYSIS	Energy	Protein	Carbohydrate	Fat	Iron
per meatball	24 kcal	3.5 g	1.3 g	0.5 g	0.21 mg

over 18 months

Makes 6 burgers

Turkey Burgers

PREHEAT BARBECUE OR GRILL

Kitchen Tip

Salsa helps to keep the lean turkey from drying out. It also adds flavor that your children will love. Moms and Dads can use a medium/hot salsa or a dash of tabasco sauce if they prefer a little spice.

1 lb	ground turkey or chicken	500 g
1/4 cup	mild salsa	50 mL
1	egg	1
3 to 4 tsp	bread crumbs	15 to 20 mL

1. In a bowl combine turkey, salsa, egg and bread crumbs; mix well. With your hands, form meat mixture into 6 balls and flatten into patties. Grill for 15 to 20 minutes or until cooked throughout.

NUTRITIONAL ANALYSIS	Energy	Protein	Carbohydrate	Fat	Iron
per burger	150 kcal	19.0 g	4.2 g	5.8 g	1.64 mg

Makes 6 1/2 cups (1.625 L)

Chili Con Carne

This chili is delicious served with grated Cheddar cheese and a dollop of sour cream on top, with some bread for dipping.

Kitchen Tip

Feel free to add whatever vegetables are handy in your kitchen. Try sautéed green and red peppers or mushrooms – or whatever your kids enjoy. Be careful if freezing this dish; once frozen and thawed, it can become quite spicy.

2 tbsp	vegetable oil	25 mL
1/2 cup	finely chopped onions	125 mL
1 lb	ground beef	500 g
1	can (28 oz [796 mL]) kidney beans, rinsed and drained	1
1	can (28 oz [796 mL]) tomatoes	1
7 oz	tomato sauce *or* canned condensed tomato soup	211 mL
1/2 to 1 tsp	granulated sugar	3 to 5 mL
1/2 tsp	chili powder	2 mL
1/2 tsp	salt	2 mL
Dash	cayenne pepper	Dash

1. In a large saucepan, heat oil over medium-high heat. Add onions and sauté until tender and translucent. Add ground beef and continue to cook until brown. Add beans, tomatoes, tomato sauce, sugar, chili powder, salt and cayenne pepper. Bring to a boil; reduce heat and simmer for 45 minutes.

NUTRITIONAL ANALYSIS	Energy	Protein	Carbohydrate	Fat	Iron
per 1/2 cup (125 mL)	201 kcal	11.5 g	15.5 g	10.6 g	2.41 mg

over 18 months

Serves 4

Makes 5 cups (1.25 L)

Kitchen Tip

Use grated Parmesan or any melting cheese for this dish.

DINNER

À la King Supper

This classic dish from a generation ago was really nothing more than a fancy way to get rid of leftovers. Well, nothing has changed. This recipe turns leftover cooked vegetables and meats into a tasty family meal, just like your mother's.

1/4 cup	butter *or* margarine	50 mL
1	medium onion, finely chopped	1
6	large mushrooms, sliced	6
3 tbsp	all-purpose flour	45 mL
2 cups	2% milk	500 mL
2 cups	cooked vegetables	500 mL
2 cups	diced cooked meat	500 mL
1/2 cup	shredded cheese (see Tip)	125 mL

Hot buttered toast or English muffins, cooked rice or baked potatoes

1. In a large saucepan, melt butter over medium-high heat. Add onion and mushrooms; cook for 5 minutes or until softened.

2. Remove pan from heat. Stir in flour, then milk. Return to heat and cook, stirring constantly, until smooth and thickened. Add vegetables, meat and cheese. Stir until cheese melts and mixture is heated.

3. Serve over toast, muffins halves, rice or potatoes.

NUTRITIONAL ANALYSIS	Energy	Protein	Carbohydrate	Fat	Iron
per 1/2 cup (125 mL)	82 kcal	6.7 g	4.8 g	4.0 g	0.46 mg

Serves 6 adults
Makes 16 baby servings

Crispy Fish

This is a delicious fish recipe that freezes well
– a great combo of cheese, spinach and fish.

PREHEAT OVEN TO 350° F (180° C)
CASSEROLE, GREASED

Half	Lemon	Half
1/2 cup	olive oil	125 mL
1	large clove garlic, minced	1
2 tbsp	dried basil	25 mL
2 cups	bread crumbs	500 mL
1/2 cup	grated Parmesan cheese	125 mL
1/4 tsp	freshly ground black pepper	1 mL
1 1/2 lbs	fillets of sole or other fish, defrosted	750 g

1. In a food processor, purée lemon and oil. Pour mixture into a skillet and heat over medium heat for 2 minutes. Add garlic and basil; sauté for about 2 minutes longer. Add bread crumbs and sauté for 3 to 4 minutes or until they are dry. Transfer mixture to a bowl. Stir in Parmesan cheese and pepper.

2. Place fish in prepared casserole. Spread topping over fish. Cover and bake in preheated oven for 20 minutes or until fish flakes easily with a fork.

NUTRITIONAL ANALYSIS	Energy	Protein	Carbohydrate	Fat	Iron
per baby serving	166 kcal	10.7 g	10.4 g	8.9 g	1.17 mg

Serves 4 adults

Makes 4 cups (1 L)

DINNER

Herbed Chicken

Kitchen Tip

If you can't find any fresh marjoram, substitute 2 tsp (10 mL) dried.

4	boneless skinless chicken breasts, cut into 1 1/2-inch (4 cm) strips	4
1/4 tsp	salt	1 mL
1/4 tsp	freshly ground black pepper	1 mL
2 tbsp	olive oil	25 mL
3 tbsp	butter *or* margarine	45 mL
1	onion, chopped	1
1 tbsp	all-purpose flour	15 mL
2 tbsp	lemon juice	25 mL
2 cups	chicken stock	500 mL
8 oz	mushrooms, quartered	250 g
2 tbsp	chopped fresh marjoram	25 mL
3	cloves garlic, crushed	3

1. Sprinkle chicken with salt and pepper. In a large frying pan, heat oil and 2 tbsp (25 mL) of the butter over medium heat. Add chicken and cook for about 4 to 5 minutes. Remove chicken to a warmed plate and set aside.

2. Reduce heat to medium. Melt remaining butter in pan. Add onion and cook for 2 minutes. Sprinkle with flour and cook, stirring constantly, for another 2 minutes. Stir in chicken stock and lemon juice. Return to medium-high heat. Add mushrooms, marjoram and garlic; cook for about 15 minutes or until sauce has been reduced to about 1 cup (250 mL). Return chicken to pan and heat through. Serve over steamed rice or noodles.

NUTRITIONAL ANALYSIS	Energy	Protein	Carbohydrate	Fat	Iron
per 1/2 cup (125 mL)	158 kcal	16.0 g	4.1 g	8.5 g	1.38 mg

Serves 4 adults

Makes 16 baby servings

Lemon Chicken

Try this zesty way to prepare chicken.
It's also delicious as leftovers – if there are any!

3 tbsp	all-purpose flour	45 mL
1/2 tsp	salt	2 mL
1/4 tsp	freshly ground black pepper	1 mL
2 tbsp	olive oil	25 mL
4	boneless skinless chicken breasts	4
1 tbsp	butter *or* margarine	15 mL
1	onion, finely chopped	1
1 cup	chicken stock	250 mL
3 tbsp	lemon juice	45 mL
1/2 tsp	ground thyme	2 mL

1. In a plastic bag, combine flour, salt and pepper. Add chicken and shake in bag to coat lightly. Remove the chicken and reserve the excess flour.

2. In a large skillet, heat oil over medium heat. Add chicken and brown both sides for about 5 minutes each. Transfer to a warm plate.

3. Melt butter in skillet. Add onion and cook for 3 to 4 minutes or until softened. Add excess flour and cook for 1 minute. Add chicken stock, lemon juice and thyme. Bring to a boil, stirring constantly.

4. Return chicken to pan. Reduce heat to medium-low and cook for 7 to 8 minutes or until chicken is tender and no longer pink inside.

NUTRITIONAL ANALYSIS	Energy	Protein	Carbohydrate	Fat	Iron
per baby serving	62 kcal	7.4 g	1.8 g	2.7 g	0.39 mg

over 18 months

Serves 6 adults
Makes 24 baby servings

Chicken-So-Good

PREHEAT OVEN TO 350° F (180° C)
LARGE CASSEROLE

Kitchen Tip

The sauce is best if made the day before. It's delicious served with rice or pasta.

6	boneless skinless chicken breasts	6
1/2 cup	all-purpose flour	125 mL
1/2 tsp	salt	2 mL
1/4 tsp	freshly ground black pepper	1 mL
2	eggs, slightly beaten	2
1 1/2 cups	crushed Special K cereal	375 mL
1/3 cup	vegetable oil	75 mL
	Sauce	
1/4 cup	vegetable oil	50 mL
2	medium onions, minced	2
2	cloves garlic, minced	2
1 1/2	green peppers, diced	1 1/2
1 cup	sliced canned mushrooms	250 mL
1 tsp	salt	5 mL
1/2 tsp	freshly ground black pepper	2 mL
1 tsp	dried oregano	5 mL
2 tsp	Worcestershire sauce	10 mL
1/4 tsp	Tabasco sauce	1 mL
1	1 can (2.8 oz [80 mL] tomato paste	1
1	1 can (28 oz [796 mL] tomato sauce	1
1/2 cup	water	125 mL
1 tbsp	lemon juice	15 mL
2 tsp	granulated sugar	10 mL

1. Place chicken between sheets of wax paper and pound until quite thin. In a bowl combine flour, salt and pepper. Dip chicken in flour mixture, then in eggs. Coat with cereal crumbs.

2. In a large skillet, heat 1/3 cup (75 mL) oil over medium-high heat. Add chicken and sauté on both sides for about 10 minutes. Transfer chicken to casserole.

3. Sauce: Add 1/4 cup (50 mL) oil to skillet. Add onions, garlic, green peppers and mushrooms; sauté for about 5 minutes. Add salt, pepper, oregano, Worcestershire sauce, tabasco sauce, tomato paste and sauce, water, lemon juice and sugar. Cover and simmer for approximately 30 minutes. Add more water if sauce appears too thick.

4. Pour sauce over chicken in casserole. Bake in preheated oven for 35 minutes.

NUTRITIONAL ANALYSIS	Energy	Protein	Carbohydrate	Fat	Iron
per baby serving	115 kcal	8.6 g	7.4 g	5.8 g	1.14 mg

over 18 months

Serves 4 adults

Makes 16 baby servings

Thai Chicken

PREHEAT OVEN TO 375° F (190° C)

BAKING DISH

Kitchen Tip

Delicious when served over rice with a favorite vegetable!

Fish sauce is available in Asian markets or in the oriental food section of large supermarkets.

1 tbsp	olive oil	15 mL
4	boneless skinless chicken breasts	4
2 tbsp	dried coriander	25 mL
2 tbsp	dried basil	25 mL
1 tbsp	dried mint	15 mL
1 tbsp	lemon juice	15 mL
2 tbsp	vegetable oil	25 mL
1 tbsp	granulated sugar	15 mL
2 tbsp	fish sauce	25 mL
3	garlic cloves, minced	3
1 tsp	grated lemon zest	5 mL
2	green onions, chopped	2

1. In a large skillet, heat oil over high heat. Add chicken and cook until browned. Set aside.

2. In a large bowl, combine coriander, basil, mint, lemon juice, oil, sugar, fish sauce, garlic, lemon zest and green onions.

3. Place chicken in marinade; refrigerate for at least 1 hour or overnight.

4. Remove chicken from marinade and place in baking dish. Bake in preheated oven for 20 minutes or until cooked through.

NUTRITIONAL ANALYSIS	Energy	Protein	Carbohydrate	Fat	Iron
per baby serving	62 kcal	7.1 g	1.6 g	3.0 g	0.69 mg

Serves 4 Adults

Makes 16 baby servings

Baked Sweet 'n' Sour Chicken

Food Safety Tip

Keep raw poultry (as well as other raw meats) away from other foods during storage and preparation. As well, keep separate cutting boards for raw meats and vegetables.

The sauce adds a sweet pungent taste to chicken served over rice. It's a taste that many children adore and, of course, so do their elders.

PREHEAT OVEN TO 350° F (180° C)

RECTANGULAR CASSEROLE, GREASED

4	boneless skinless chicken breasts (half breasts)	4
1/2 cup	tomato sauce	125 mL
Half	small onion, finely chopped	Half
3 tbsp	brown sugar	45 mL
2 tbsp	cider vinegar	25 mL
1/2 cup	crushed pineapple, with juice	125 mL
1	clove garlic, mashed	1
	Cooked rice	
	Chopped fresh parsley	

1. Place chicken breasts in prepared casserole.

2. In a small bowl, combine tomato sauce, onion, sugar, vinegar, pineapple (with juice) and garlic; spoon over chicken. Bake in preheated oven for 45 minutes or until chicken is no longer pink and juices run clear.

3. Serve chicken and sauce over cooked rice sprinkled with parsley.

NUTRITIONAL ANALYSIS	Energy	Protein	Carbohydrate	Fat	Iron
per baby serving	52 kcal	6.8 g	4.2 g	0.8 g	1.19 mg

over 18 months

Serves 4 adults

Makes 16 baby servings

Chicken Pad Thai

Kitchen Tips

For an authentic finish to this dish, and where there is no danger of allergy, sprinkle 4 tbsp (60 mL) chopped unsalted peanuts over dish just before serving.

Fish sauce is available in Asian markets or in the oriental food section of large supermarkets.

7 oz	wide rice stick noodles	200 g
2/3 cup	chicken stock	150 mL
1/3 cup	ketchup	75 mL
1/4 cup	fish sauce (see Tip)	50 mL
2 tbsp	granulated sugar	25 mL
2 tbsp	cornstarch	25 mL
2 tbsp	lime juice	25 mL
1 tsp	hot pepper sauce	5 mL
4 tsp	vegetable oil, divided	20 mL
2	eggs, beaten	2
1 lb	boneless skinless chicken breasts cut into thin strips	500 g
4	carrots, julienned	4
1	red pepper bell pepper, thinly sliced	1
2	garlic cloves, minced	2
1 tbsp	minced ginger root	15 mL
2 cups	bean sprouts	500 mL
2	green onions, chopped	2

1. In a large pot, soak noodles in warm water to cover for 30 minutes. Drain.

2. In a small bowl, combine chicken stock, ketchup, fish sauce, sugar, cornstarch, lime juice and hot pepper sauce. Mix well and set aside.

3. In a large nonstick skillet or wok, heat 2 tsp (10 mL) of the oil over medium–high heat. Add eggs and scramble for about 2 to 3 minutes. Transfer to a plate and set aside.

4. Heat remaining oil in same skillet or wok. Add chicken and stir-fry until browned; transfer to a plate and set aside. Add carrots, red pepper, garlic and ginger; stir-fry for about 5 minutes. Add noodles and stir-fry for another 2 minutes.

5. Return chicken to wok. Stir in reserved sauce and cook for about 5 minutes or until chicken is thoroughly cooked. Toss in egg mixture, bean sprouts and green onions; cook until warmed throughout.

NUTRITIONAL ANALYSIS	Energy	Protein	Carbohydrate	Fat	Iron
per baby serving	125 kcal	12.4 g	10.7 g	3.8 g	1.14 mg

Makes 2 cups (500 mL)

DINNER

Chicken Stir-Fry

The infants who tested this stir-fry showed great interest in its color as well as its flavor. Their parents liked it too!

Kitchen Tip

Cooked white or brown rice is the perfect complement to this fast stir-fry recipe. The rice will cook in about 15 minutes, so start it just before starting to cook the stir-fry.

Food Safety Tip

If you are using frozen chicken breasts, the safest way to thaw them (or any other frozen meats) is in the refrigerator. Allow 6 to 9 hours per lb (14 to 20 hours per kg). Leave chicken in its freezer wrapper on a tray or plate on the bottom shelf. Never allow meat to thaw at room temperature. If you do, bacteria can grow on the surface of the meat, even while the inside remains frozen.

1 tbsp	hoisin sauce	15 mL
1 tbsp	soy sauce	15 mL
2 tsp	rice vinegar *or* white vinegar	10 mL
1/2 tsp	sesame oil	2 mL
Half	red bell pepper, cut into large chunks	Half
6	medium mushrooms, cut into large chunks	6
1 cup	small broccoli florets	250 mL
2	boneless skinless chicken breasts (half breasts), cut into chunks	2
1 tbsp	vegetable oil	15 mL
2 cups	bean sprouts	500 mL

1. In a bowl combine hoisin and soy sauce, vinegar and sesame oil. Add red pepper, mushrooms and broccoli; toss to coat. Set aside.

2. In a wok or large nonstick skillet, heat oil over medium-high heat. Add chicken and cook, stirring constantly, for 3 minutes or until no longer pink. Add vegetable mixture; cover and steam for 5 minutes. Stir in bean sprouts; cover and steam for 2 minutes.

NUTRITIONAL ANALYSIS	Energy	Protein	Carbohydrate	Fat	Iron
per 1/2 cup (125 mL)	139 kcal	17.3 g	7.5 g	5.0 g	1.78 mg

Beef Stroganoff

Serves 4 adults
Makes 16 baby servings
or 8 cups (2 L)

Kitchen Tip

Any kind of boneless beef you would like to use will work. Slicing the beef into thin strips will help the beef to cook faster and will make it easier for your children to enjoy.

1/4 cup	butter *or* margarine, divided	50 mL
2	small onions, chopped	2
10	mushrooms, sliced	10
1 lb	beef filet (tenderloin), cut across the grain into thin strips	500 g
3	tomatoes, peeled and diced	3
	Salt and freshly ground black pepper to taste	
1 cup	sour cream	250 mL
2 cups	hot cooked noodles	500 mL

1. In a large skillet, melt 1 tbsp (15 mL) of the butter over medium-high heat. Add onions and cook for 5 minutes. Remove onions to a bowl and set aside.

2. Add mushroom slices and cook for 4 minutes. Remove and set aside.

3. Add remaining butter to skillet. Increase heat to high. Add beef and cook for 3 minutes. Return vegetables to skillet. Season to taste with salt and the pepper. Stir in sour cream. Heat just until mixture begins to simmer. Serve over noodles.

NUTRITIONAL ANALYSIS	Energy	Protein	Carbohydrate	Fat	Iron
per 1/2 cup (125 mL)	124 kcal	8.3 g	7.2 g	6.9 g	1.28 mg

over 18 months

Serves 8 adults

Makes 16 baby servings

DINNER

Beef Sour Cream Noodle Bake

Kitchen Tips

If you use spaghetti sauce instead of plain tomato sauce, you may not need to add the basil and oregano unless extra spice is desired.

Cooked beef mixture may be prepared to the end of Step 1 and frozen, or used at once in the casserole recipe.

If eating one casserole, which is sufficient for 4, cover and freeze the second one for later use.

Cooked vegetables may be added if desired.

This excellent make-ahead casserole is economical to prepare and freeze well for later use. Make it in one casserole for a crowd or large family. Noodles and cheese make this dish attractive to younger family members. It also sticks together for easy eating.

PREHEAT OVEN TO 350° F (180° C)

TWO 4-CUP (1 L) CASSEROLES, GREASED

1 lb	lean or medium ground beef	500 g
1	medium onion, finely chopped	1
2	cloves garlic, minced	2
1 cup	tomato sauce *or* spaghetti sauce	250 mL
1 tsp	dried basil (see Tip)	5 mL
1 tsp	dried oregano (see Tip)	5 mL
1/4 tsp	salt	1 mL
1/4 tsp	freshly ground black pepper	1 mL
2 cups	uncooked broad egg noodles	500 mL
1 cup	2% cottage cheese	250 mL
1 cup	sour cream	250 mL
3/4 cup	shredded mozzarella or mild Cheddar cheese	175 mL

1. In a large nonstick skillet, cook beef, onion and garlic until beef is no longer pink; drain excess fat. Add tomato sauce and seasonings. Bring to a boil. Reduce heat to low and cook for 5 minutes.

2. Meanwhile, in a large saucepan, cook noodles in boiling water according to package directions or until tender but firm. Drain. Add cottage cheese and sour cream; stir to combine.

3. Spoon one-quarter of noodle mixture into pre-
    pared casseroles. Cover each with one-quarter of
    ground beef mixture; repeat layers. Divide cheese
    over top of each casserole. Bake, uncovered, for
    35 minutes or until thoroughly heated.

NUTRITIONAL ANALYSIS	Energy	Protein	Carbohydrate	Fat	Iron
per baby serving	172 kcal	12.4 g	8.1 g	9.9 g	1.04 mg

over 18 months

Makes 9 cups (2.25 L)

Beef and Vegetable Stew

2 tbsp	all-purpose flour	25 mL
1/4 tsp	salt	1 mL
Dash	freshly ground black pepper	Dash
1 1/4 lbs	stewing beef, cut into bite-size cubes	625 g
2 tbsp	butter *or* margarine	25 mL
1	onion, chopped	1
2 2/3 cups	beef stock	650 mL
3	carrots, peeled and sliced	3
3	stalks celery, chopped	3
1 cup	sliced mushrooms	250 mL
1	can (28oz [796 mL]) chopped tomatoes	1

1. In a small bowl, stir together flour, salt and pepper. Dredge beef in flour. Shake off any excess and transfer to a plate.

2. In a large saucepan, melt butter over medium-high heat. Add beef and onion; cook for about 2 minutes or until meat is browned and onion has softened. Stir in stock slowly and bring to a boil; cook, stirring constantly, until thick. Add carrots, celery, mushrooms and tomatoes; cover and let simmer for 2 to 2 1/2 hours.

NUTRITIONAL ANALYSIS	Energy	Protein	Carbohydrate	Fat	Iron
per 1/2 cup (125 mL)	84 kcal	8.3 g	4.6 g	3.6 g	1.17 mg

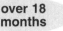

over 18 months

Serves 4

Pork Chops in Creamy Herb Sauce

Lean and tender pork chops are cooked in a pineapple-herb sauce, which keeps them moist and flavorful.

1 tbsp	vegetable oil	15 mL
4	boneless lean pork chops	4
1	small onion, sliced	1
1/2 cup	pineapple juice	125 mL
1/2 tsp	dried tarragon	2 mL
1/2 tsp	dried thyme	2 mL
1	large apple, cut into eighths	1
1/2 cup	sour cream	125 mL
1 tbsp	all-purpose flour	15 mL

1. In a skillet just large enough to hold chops, heat oil over medium–high heat. Brown chops on each side. Remove to a warm plate. Add onion and sauté for 3 minutes. Add pineapple juice, tarragon and thyme.

2. Return chops to skillet. Bring to a boil. Reduce heat, cover and cook for 15 minutes or until meat is tender. Add apple during last 5 minutes of cooking.

3. Remove meat, apple and onion to a warm platter. Boil remaining liquid to reduce slightly.

4. In a small bowl, whisk together sour cream and flour. Stir into boiling liquid, stirring constantly until thickened. Pour sauce over chops and serve. Cut infant's portion into small pieces.

NUTRITIONAL ANALYSIS	Energy	Protein	Carbohydrate	Fat	Iron
per chop	279 kcal	22.9 g	13.0 g	14.9 g	1.20 mg

over 18 months

Serves 6
Makes 6 cups (1.5 L)

Food Safety Tip

Take care that juices from any meats or poultry do not drip onto other foods. Keep raw meats and poultry separate from cooked meats or cold cuts in the refrigerator. This will prevent cross-contamination.

DINNER

Homestyle Oven Pork and Barley Stew

Busy parents love stews because once the preparation is complete, cooking continues without any further work. And they are great for children. It's easy to adjust portions for their smaller appetites and the individual pieces of the stew are easy for them to handle.

PREHEAT OVEN TO 375° F (190° C)

LARGE ROASTING PAN

1/4 cup	all-purpose flour	50 mL
1/2 tsp	salt	2 mL
1/2 tsp	dried thyme	2 mL
1 1/4 lbs	lean pork shoulder, trimmed of all visible fat and cut into cubes	625 g
2 tbsp	vegetable oil	25 mL
1 cup	apple juice	250 mL
1/2 cup	pearl barley	125 mL
4	carrots, peeled and cut into pieces	4
2	onions, cut into wedges	2
2	cloves garlic, finely chopped	2
3	strips orange zest	3
1	bay leaf	1
1 cup	water (approximate)	250 mL

1. In a plastic bag, combine flour, salt and thyme. Add pork cubes and toss to coat. Remove pork; reserve excess flour.

2. Add oil to large roasting pan. Stir in floured pork. Bake, uncovered, in preheated oven for 20 minutes; stir once.

3. Reduce oven temperature to 350°F (180°C). In a
    bowl, stir together apple juice and reserved flour;
    pour over meat. Add barley, carrots, onions, garlic,
    orange zest and bay leaf. Bake, covered, for
    45 minutes or until pork and barley are tender.
    (Stir occasionally to check thickness of sauce; add
    water as mixture thickens.)

4. Remove orange zest and bay leaf before serving.

NUTRITIONAL ANALYSIS	Energy	Protein	Carbohydrate	Fat	Iron
per 1/2 cup (125 mL)	149 kcal	12.0 g	14.0 g	4.9 g	1.08 mg

over 18 months

Makes 6 cups (1.5 L)

Kitchen Tip

Stews freeze well, so why not double the recipe?

Pork Stew with Vegetables

Stew always gives a wonderful lift to the day. We've noticed that most young family members enjoy stew as much as their older relatives.

2 tsp	vegetable oil	10 mL
1 lb	lean pork shoulder, trimmed of all visible fat and cut into small cubes	500 g
1	medium onion, finely chopped	1
1	medium cooking apple, cored and chopped	1
2	medium tomatoes, chopped	2
1/4 cup	apple juice	50 mL
1/4 cup	water	50 mL
1/4 tsp	ground cinnamon	1 mL
1/4 tsp	curry powder	1 mL
1/4 tsp	salt	1 mL
1	bay leaf	1
2	large potatoes, diced	2

1. In a large skillet, heat oil over medium–high heat. Add pork and onion; cook for about 10 minutes or until golden. Add apple, tomatoes, apple juice, water, cinnamon, curry powder, salt and bay leaf. Cover, reduce heat and simmer for about 1 hour or until pork is tender.

2. Meanwhile, in a small saucepan, bring water to a boil. Add potatoes and cook for 15 minutes or until tender. Mash or serve in pieces.

3. Remove bay leaf from stew before serving over potato.

NUTRITIONAL ANALYSIS	Energy	Protein	Carbohydrate	Fat	Iron
per 1/2 cup (125 mL)	134 kcal	12.8 g	7.3 g	5.8 g	0.83 mg

Snacks

ABCDEFGHIJKLMNOPQRSTUVWXYZ

8 to 12 months

Makes 4 cups (1 L)

Homemade Yogurt

KITCHEN THERMOMETER

Kitchen Tip

For this recipe to work, all bowls, pots and utensils must be very clean.

Serve yogurt over fruit or enjoy on its own.

4 cups	2% milk	1 L
1/2 cup	plain yogurt	125 mL

1. In a large heavy saucepan, heat milk slowly, stirring occasionally, until it reaches 180° F (45° C). Transfer to a clean bowl. Let milk cool to 113° F (45° C).

2. In a small cup, mix yogurt with 1/4 cup (50 mL) of the warm milk. Stir back into warmed milk. Cover bowl and wrap in tea towels to ensure mixture cools as slowly as possible. Let sit undisturbed for a minimum of 5 hours, then refrigerate. Keeps refrigerated for up to 1 week.

NUTRITIONAL ANALYSIS per 1/4 cup (50 mL)	Energy	Protein	Carbohydrate	Fat	Iron
	45 kcal	2.4 g	3.4 g	2.4 g	0.04 mg

8 to 12 months

Makes about 1 cup (250 mL)

Yogurt Cheese

Kitchen Tip

This soft cheese makes a great dip. Combine with French onion soup mix and serve with veggies.

If you don't have cheesecloth, a coffee filter will also work.

Nutrition Note

Because the composition of yogurt changes when it is drained, a nutritional analysis is not supplied with this recipe. Keep in mind that calories will increase with higher percentages of milk fat.

2 cups	plain yogurt	500 mL

1. Line a sieve with cheesecloth. Add yogurt and let drain for approximately 30 minutes.

2. Tie a knot in the top of cheesecloth with a wooden spoon. Suspend over a large bowl and keep overnight in the refrigerator.

3. Untie cheesecloth and remove cheese. Keep chilled until ready to serve.

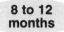

8 to 12 months

Makes 12

Chapati
(Indian Bread)

Serving Suggestion

This bread is great with curried beef or chicken for lunch or dinner, or with jam and cream cheese for breakfast.

1 1/2 cups	whole wheat flour	375 mL
3/4 cup	all-purpose flour	175 mL
1/4 tsp	salt	1 mL
1 cup	water	250 mL

Vegetable oil for frying

1. In a bowl combine all-purpose flour, whole wheat flour and salt. Add water in small amounts, mixing until the dough comes together in a ball. Knead dough for 5 minutes; let rest under a damp tea towel for about 30 minutes.

2. Divide dough into 12 pieces. Knead each piece briefly. Roll into flat circles about 5 inches (12.5 cm) in diameter.

3. In a large frying pan, heat oil over medium-high heat. Add chapati and cook one side, turning when bread puffs up. Cook other side and transfer to a plate.

NUTRITIONAL ANALYSIS	Energy	Protein	Carbohydrate	Fat	Iron
per slice	83 kcal	3.0 g	17.5 g	0.4 g	0.85 mg

12 to 18 months

Makes 1/4 cup (50 mL)

Citrus Yogurt Fruit Dip

Fussy little appetites can be enticed into trying new fruits with this yogurt dip. Children enjoy the fun of dipping – and this is about as nutritious as a snack can get.

Kitchen Tip

For a slightly sweeter – although higher-fat – version of this dip, substitute sour cream for yogurt.

This recipe is easily doubled.

1/4 cup	plain yogurt (see Tip)	50 mL
1 tsp	frozen orange juice concentrate, thawed	5 mL
Pinch	granulated sugar	
Pinch	ground ginger	Pinch
Pinch	ground nutmeg	Pinch

Fruit, such as banana chunks, orange or mandarin segments, seedless grapes cut in half, cantaloupe or honeydew chunks, apple or pear slices, strawberry slices

1. In a small bowl, combine yogurt, orange juice, sugar, ginger and nutmeg; stir well. For best flavor, chill for a short time in the refrigerator. Serve with fruit pieces for dipping.

NUTRITIONAL ANALYSIS	Energy	Protein	Carbohydrate	Fat	Iron
per 1 tbsp (15 mL)	14 kcal	0.6 g	1.9 g	0.5 g	0.02 mg

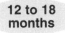

12 to 18 months

Makes 2 1/3 cups (575 mL)

Spinach Cottage Cheese Dip

Kitchen Tip

Return any remaining dip to the refrigerator for up to 4 days.

Few can resist this nutritious and eye-pleasing dip (and the fun of dipping). In time, they may even decide they like their spinach "straight up." Use vegetables or corn tortilla chips as dippers.

1	pkg (10 oz) [284 g]) frozen chopped spinach, thawed, excess liquid squeezed out	1
1 cup	cottage cheese	250 mL
1	small clove garlic	1
1 cup	sour cream	250 mL
Dash	Tabasco sauce	Dash
1/8 tsp	salt	0.5 mL

1. In a food processor, combine spinach, cottage cheese and garlic; process with on/off turns until fairly smooth. Add sour cream, Tabasco sauce and salt; process to blend.

2. Transfer dip to a bowl; cover and refrigerate for several hours or overnight to allow flavors to develop.

NUTRITIONAL ANALYSIS	Energy	Protein	Carbohydrate	Fat	Iron
per 1 tbsp (15 mL)	18 kcal	1.2 g	0.7 g	1.2 g	0.23 mg

12 to 18 months

SNACKS

Red Pepper Dip

Makes 3/4 cup (175 mL)

Everybody likes to dip. And the smoky-sweet taste of roasted red peppers in this sour-cream-based dip is irresistible. Torn pieces of pita bread, bread sticks and fresh vegetables make excellent dippers.

Kitchen Tip

If you have time, roast your own peppers under a broiler or on a barbecue grill, then remove skin and seeds. This is especially worthwhile when peppers are in season. Roasted peppers can be frozen for later use.

1/2 cup	drained bottled roasted red peppers (see Tip)	125 mL
1/4 cup	sour cream	50 mL
2 tbsp	mayonnaise	25 mL
1 tsp	lemon juice	5 mL
1/2 tsp	ground oregano	2 mL
Pinch	granulated sugar	Pinch
Pinch	salt	Pinch

1. In a food processor or blender, combine red peppers, sour cream, mayonnaise and lemon juice; purée until smooth. Stir in oregano, sugar and salt. Spoon into a container with a tight-fitting lid. Refrigerate until ready to serve.

NUTRITIONAL ANALYSIS	Energy	Protein	Carbohydrate	Fat	Iron
per 1 tbsp (15 mL)	23 kcal	0.3 g	0.8 g	2.2 g	0.12 mg

12 to 18
months

Makes 1 1/2 cups (375 mL)

Hummus
(Chickpea Dip)

Kitchen Tips

To peel chickpeas, squeeze them gently and the thin skin will slide off. This will give your hummus a smoother texture. But if you're short of time, leave the skins on.

Tahini is sesame seed paste. It can be found in Middle Eastern grocery stores or in some large supermarkets.

3 tbsp	tahini	45 mL
2 tbsp	cold water	25 mL
	Juice of 1 lemon	
1	can (19 oz [540 mL]) chickpeas, peeled (see Tip)	1
1	clove garlic, minced	1

1. In a small bowl, combine tahini with cold water, stirring until tahini turns white. Transfer paste to food processor along with chickpeas; blend until mixed. Add lemon juice and garlic; purée to desired consistency, adding more water as necessary. Serve with pita bread.

NUTRITIONAL ANALYSIS	Energy	Protein	Carbohydrate	Fat	Iron
per tbsp (15 mL)	40 kcal	2.0 g	5.6 g	1.4 g	0.66 mg

12 to 18 months

Makes 4 cups (1 L)

Tangy Salsa

Kitchen Tip

Avocado adds calories and is a great source of monounsaturated fat.

Stores refrigerated for 2 to 3 days.

4	tomatoes, chopped and seeded	4
Half	onion, chopped	Half
1/2 cup	chopped peeled avocado	125 mL
1/4 cup	chopped fresh coriander	50 mL
2 tbsp	vegetable oil	25 mL
2 tbsp	lime juice	25 mL
Pinch	salt	Pinch
Pinch	freshly ground black pepper	Pinch

1. In a large bowl, mix together all the ingredients. Let sit for about 1 hour to develop flavors before serving.

NUTRITIONAL ANALYSIS	Energy	Protein	Carbohydrate	Fat	Iron
per 1/4 cup (50 mL)	33 kcal	0.5 g	2.4 g	2.7 g	0.26 mg

12 to 18 months

Frozen Fruit Pops

Makes 1 cup (250 mL)
or 4 pops

This frozen yogurt snack is brimming with nutrition. .

Food Safety Tip

Honey should only be given to children who are over 1 year of age. For younger children, replace honey in this recipe with granulated sugar.

1 cup	sliced strawberries or cubed cantaloupe	250 mL
1/2 cup	plain yogurt	125 mL
2 tbsp	instant skim milk powder	25 mL
2 tbsp	liquid honey (see Tip)	25 mL
1/2 cup	evaporated milk	125 mL

1. In a food processor or blender, combine fruit, yogurt, milk powder and honey; process until smooth. Blend in milk.

2. Spoon mixture into small molds or paper cups. Freeze until pops are almost solid; insert a plastic spoon or tongue depressor into the center of each mold. Return to freezer. When frozen, store in a sealed plastic bag until ready to serve.

NUTRITIONAL ANALYSIS	Energy	Protein	Carbohydrate	Fat	Iron
per fruit pop	96 kcal	4.5 g	16.3 g	1.9 g	0.29 mg

Makes 2 1/2 cups (625 mL)

Cereal Snack

Here's a simplified "nuts and bolts" snack that children love. (They especially enjoy feeding themselves with the small, easily handled pieces.) It's quick to make and provides more food energy than the cereal alone.

1 tbsp	margarine *or* butter	15 mL
1 1/2 cups	Cheerios-type oat cereal	375 mL
1/2 cup	pretzels, broken	125 mL
1/2 cup	finely chopped raisins	125 mL

1. In a large nonstick skillet, melt margarine over medium-low heat. Add cereal and cook, stirring constantly, for 5 minutes. Remove from heat and allow to cool. Stir in pretzels and raisins. Store in an airtight container.

NUTRITIONAL ANALYSIS	Energy	Protein	Carbohydrate	Fat	Iron
per 1/4 cup (50 mL)	91 kcal	1.8 g	17.2 g	2.0 g	0.81 mg

Makes 24 cookies

French Biscuits

PREHEAT OVEN TO 375° F (190° C)

BAKING SHEET

Kitchen Tip

These basic sugar cookies are quick and easy to make using ingredients that are always on hand. Keep an eye on them, since they can burn very quickly.

2/3 cup	butter *or* margarine	150 mL
2/3 cup	all-purpose flour	150 mL
1/3 cup	granulated sugar	75 mL

1. In a large bowl with an electric mixer, blend together butter, flour and sugar. Drop small dollops onto cookie sheet. Bake in preheated oven for 7 to 10 minutes or until golden brown.

NUTRITIONAL ANALYSIS	Energy	Protein	Carbohydrate	Fat	Iron
per cookie	65 kcal	0.4 g	5.1 g	4.9 g	0.13 mg

12 to 18 months

Makes 16

Herbed Breadsticks

Kitchen Tip

Keep unbaked bread sticks in the freezer, ready to pull out and bake at a moment's notice. Or bake them all at once for a crowd.

Breadsticks are easy to hold, making them ideal for young children who are learning to feed themselves. Adults enjoy them, too, as an accompaniment to soup or chili.

PREHEAT OVEN TO 425° F (220° C)
NONSTICK BAKING SHEET

1	long thin baguette	1
1/4 cup	butter or margarine, softened	25 mL
2 tsp	chopped fresh parsley	10 mL
1/4 tsp	ground basil	1 mL
1	small clove garlic, crushed (optional)	1

1. Cut baguette crosswise into quarters. Cut each quarter lengthwise into quarters to form 16 bread sticks.

2. In a small bowl, combine butter, parsley, basil and garlic, if using. Spread mixture thinly over cut sides of bread sticks. Place sticks in a single layer on baking sheet.

3. Bake in preheated oven for 10 minutes or until lightly toasted. Serve immediately, allowing child's portion to cool enough for safe and easy handling.

NUTRITIONAL ANALYSIS	Energy	Protein	Carbohydrate	Fat	Iron
per breadstick	67 kcal	1.9 g	8.5 g	2.9 g	0.55 mg

12 to 18 months

Makes one 12-slice loaf

Five-Grain Loaf

Kitchen Tips

Five-grain cereal can be found in the bulk-food section of many supermarkets or in health food stores. If you can't find any, use Red River cereal, which is a 3-grain cereal of cracked wheat, cracked rye and flax.

Use dried fruit such as apricots, raisins, dates, prunes or pineapple.

Cut loaf into individual slices, wrap well and freeze until needed.

Five-grain cereal adds texture, flavor and great nutrients to this quick bread. Serve for dessert with a piece of fresh fruit.

PREHEAT OVEN TO 350° F (180° C)

9- BY 5-INCH (2 L) LOAF PAN, GREASED

1 cup	5-grain cereal (see Tip)	250 mL
1 1/2 cups	buttermilk	375 mL
1	egg	1
1/4 cup	packed brown sugar	50 mL
1/4 cup	vegetable oil	50 mL
2 cups	all-purpose flour	500 mL
1/4 cup	chopped dried fruit (see Tip)	50 mL
1 tsp	baking powder	5 mL
1 tsp	baking soda	5 mL
1 tsp	ground cinnamon	5 mL
1/4 tsp	salt	1 mL

1. In a small bowl, combine cereal and buttermilk. Let stand for 5 minutes. Add egg, sugar and oil; mix well.

2. In a large bowl, combine flour, fruit, baking powder, baking soda, cinnamon and salt. Add cereal mixture to flour mixture. Stir just until dry ingredients are moistened.

3. Spoon batter into prepared loaf pan. Bake in preheated oven for 45 minutes or until a cake taster inserted in center comes out clean. Cool on a wire rack before cutting into slices.

NUTRITIONAL ANALYSIS	Energy	Protein	Carbohydrate	Fat	Iron
per slice	154 kcal	3.9 g	23.7 g	4.8 g	1.23 mg

12 to 18 months

Makes 36 cookies

Soft Cranberry Banana Cookies

Variation

For a peanut flavored version of these cookies – and where there is no danger of nut allergy – replace the butter or margarine with peanut butter.

Mashed bananas and rolled oats give body, taste, texture and nutritive value to these soft cookies. They are just the thing for a children's snack or to finish a family meal.

PREHEAT OVEN TO 350° F (180° C)

BAKING SHEETS, GREASED

1/2 cup	finely chopped dried cranberries (optional)	125 mL
1	ripe medium banana, mashed	1
1/3 cup	butter *or* margarine (see Tip)	75 mL
1/4 cup	apple juice	50 mL
1	egg	1
1/2 tsp	vanilla extract	2 mL
1 cup	rolled oats	250 mL
1/2 cup	all-purpose flour	125 mL
1/4 cup	packed brown sugar	50 mL
1 tsp	baking soda	5 mL

1. In a bowl stir together cranberries (if using), banana, butter, apple juice, egg and vanilla; mix until smooth. Stir in rolled oats, flour, sugar and baking soda; blend well.

2. Drop by spoonfuls onto baking pans; flatten with a fork. Bake in preheated oven for 10 minutes or until lightly browned. Cool on a wire rack before storing in a tightly closed container.

NUTRITIONAL ANALYSIS	Energy	Protein	Carbohydrate	Fat	Iron
per cookie	43 kcal	0.8 g	5.5 g	2.0 g	0.56 mg

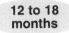

12 to 18 months

Makes about 45 cookies

Carrot Cookies

Kitchen Tip

Spread plain butter icing between 2 cookies to make a sandwich.

These cookies freeze well.

These drop cookies have an old-fashioned taste that will remind you of your grandmother's sugar cookies. The difference is the carrots, which give the cookies colorful eye appeal and vitamin A. These cookies are sized just right for little hands.

PREHEAT OVEN TO 400° F (200° C)

BAKING SHEETS, UNGREASED

1/2 cup	butter *or* margarine	125 mL
1 cup	packed brown sugar	250 mL
1	egg	1
1 cup	finely shredded carrots (about 2 medium)	250 mL
1 1/2 cups	all-purpose flour	375 mL
1 cup	whole wheat flour	250 mL
1 tsp	ground cinnamon	5 mL
1 tsp	baking powder	5 mL
1/2 tsp	ground nutmeg	2 mL
1/2 tsp	salt	2 mL

1. In a large bowl with an electric mixer, cream together butter with sugar until light and fluffy. Beat in egg and carrots.

2. In another bowl, combine flours, cinnamon, baking powder, nutmeg and salt. Gradually stir into creamed mixture, blending well after each addition.

3. Drop cookies on baking sheets; press down with a moistened fork. Bake in preheated oven for 15 minutes or until cookies are golden and crisp. Allow cookies to cool on wire racks.

NUTRITIONAL ANALYSIS	Energy	Protein	Carbohydrate	Fat	Iron
per cookie	67 kcal	1.0 g	10.6 g	2.4 g	0.49 mg

12 to 18 months

Makes 30

Oat and Rice Crisp Cookies

Serve these small cookies (just right for little hands) with a piece of fresh fruit at snacking time. Rolled oats add a nutritional variation on the more common rice cereal cookie.

PREHEAT OVEN TO 350° F (180° C)

NONSTICK BAKING SHEETS

1/4 cup	vegetable oil	50 mL
1/2 cup	packed brown sugar	125 mL
1	egg	1
2 tbsp	corn syrup	25 mL
1/2 tsp	vanilla extract	2 mL
1 cup	all-purpose flour	250 mL
1/4 cup	skim milk powder	50 mL
1/4 tsp	salt	1 mL
1/4 tsp	baking soda	1 mL
3/4 cup	rolled oats	175 mL
1/2 cup	crisp rice cereal	125 mL

1. In a large bowl with an electric mixer, combine oil, brown sugar, egg, corn syrup and vanilla; beat until light and fluffy.

2. In another bowl, combine flour, skim milk powder, salt and baking soda. Gradually stir into creamed mixture; mix well.

3. Stir in rolled oats and cereal. Drop dough, by spoonfuls, 2 inches (5 cm) apart on cookie sheets. Bake in preheated oven for 10 minutes or until cookies are golden brown. Cool on wire rack before storing in an airtight container.

NUTRITIONAL ANALYSIS	Energy	Protein	Carbohydrate	Fat	Iron
per cookie	62 kcal	1.3 g	10.1 g	1.9 g	0.54 mg

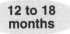

12 to 18 months

Makes 40 cookies

Apple Oatmeal Cookies

PREHEAT OVEN TO 375° F (190° C)

BAKING SHEETS, GREASED

1 cup	all-purpose flour	250 mL
1 1/4 tsp	ground cinnamon	6 mL
1/2 tsp	salt	2 mL
1/4 tsp	baking soda	1 mL
1/4 tsp	ground nutmeg	1 mL
3/4 cup	shortening	175 mL
1 1/4 cups	lightly packed brown sugar	300 mL
1	egg	1
1/4 cup	milk	50 mL
1 1/2 tsp	vanilla extract	7 mL
3 cups	rolled oats	750 mL
1 cup	finely chopped peeled apples	250 mL
1 cup	finely chopped raisins (optional)	250 mL

1. In a large bowl, combine flour, cinnamon, salt, baking soda and nutmeg.

2. In another large bowl with an electric mixer, combine shortening, brown sugar, egg, milk and vanilla; cream together until smooth. Add flour mixture with mixer on low speed, just until blended. Stir in oats, apples and raisins, if using.

3. Drop dough by spoonfuls onto prepared baking sheets. Bake for 12 minutes, or until golden brown.

NUTRITIONAL ANALYSIS	Energy	Protein	Carbohydrate	Fat	Iron
per cookie	103 kcal	1.6 g	14.8 g	4.4 g	0.68 mg

12 to 18 months

Makes one 16-slice cake

Snacking Cake

Kitchen Tip

If using a nonstick pan, there's no need to grease the cake pan.

This cake makes a nice change from cookies and milk at snack time.
Kids love it!

PREHEAT OVEN TO 375° F (190° C)

8- OR 9-INCH (20 OR 23 CM) CAKE PAN, GREASED AND FLOURED

1 1/3 cups	all-purpose flour	325 mL
2 1/2 tsp	baking powder	12 mL
1/2 cup	granulated sugar	125 mL
1/2 tsp	salt	2 mL
1/4 cup	vegetable oil	50 mL
1	egg, beaten	1
1/2 tsp	vanilla extract	2 mL
3/4 cup	2% milk	175 mL
Streusel Topping		
1/4 cup	packed brown sugar	50 mL
2 tbsp	all-purpose flour	25 mL
1 to 2 tsp	ground cinnamon	5 to 10 mL
1 tbsp	butter *or* margarine	15 mL

1. In a bowl combine flour, baking powder, sugar and salt. Make a well or depression in the center.

2. In a small bowl, combine oil, egg, vanilla and milk. Pour into well in dry ingredients; mix just until blended. Pour into prepared cake pan.

3. Streusel topping: In a bowl combine brown sugar, 2 tbsp (25 mL) flour and cinnamon. Work in butter to make a crumbly topping. Sprinkle over batter and bake in preheated oven for 30 to 35 minutes or until a toothpick inserted in the center comes out clean.

NUTRITIONAL ANALYSIS	Energy	Protein	Carbohydrate	Fat	Iron
per slice	120 kcal	2.0 g	18.5 g	4.3 g	0.66 mg

12 to 18 months

Apple Loaf

Makes one 16-slice loaf

This loaf is really a quick bread – leavened with baking powder and soda rather than yeast. You can also think of it as a large muffin made in a loaf pan. Apples give it a delightfully fresh taste and moist texture that appeals to all ages.

PREHEAT OVEN TO 350° F (180° C)

9- BY 5-INCH (2 L) LOAF PAN, GREASED

1/3 cup	butter *or* margarine	75 mL
1 cup	granulated sugar	250 mL
1	egg	1
1 tsp	vanilla extract	5 mL
1 tsp	grated orange zest	5 mL
2 cups	all-purpose flour	500 mL
1 tsp	baking powder	5 mL
1 tsp	ground cinnamon	5 mL
1/2 tsp	baking soda	2 mL
1/2 tsp	salt	2 mL
1/3 cup	fresh orange juice	75 mL
1 cup	finely chopped apple (about 1 large)	250 mL

1. In a large bowl with an electric mixer, cream butter until light and fluffy. Gradually add sugar, egg, vanilla and orange zest; beat until smooth.

2. In another bowl, sift together flour, baking powder, cinnamon, baking soda and salt. Add dry ingredients to creamed mixture alternately with orange juice; stir after each addition. Fold in apples.

3. Spoon batter into prepared loaf pan. Bake in preheated oven for 50 minutes or until a cake tester inserted in center comes out clean.

NUTRITIONAL ANALYSIS	Energy	Protein	Carbohydrate	Fat	Iron
per slice	157 kcal	2.2 g	27.9 g	4.2 g	0.80 mg

over 18 months

SNACKS

Avocado Dip

Makes 1 1/2 cups (375 mL)

Children are especially fond of avocados – perhaps because of their mushy consistency, as well as their great tropical flavor.

Kitchen Tip

Avocado discolors quickly, so make this dip only a short time before serving. Brush cut side of unused avocado with lemon juice, cover with plastic wrap and refrigerate. (Even with this treatment, however, the avocado will become browned; this can be cut off before use.)

Buy ripe avocados that yield to gentle palm pressure, are unblemished and heavy for their size.

1	ripe medium avocado, peeled (see Tip)	1
2 tsp	lemon juice	10 mL
1/4 cup	finely chopped onion	50 mL
1/4 tsp	salt	1 mL
Pinch	freshly ground black pepper	Pinch
1/4 cup	sour cream	50 mL
	Crisp corn tortillas	

1. In a bowl with a fork, mash avocado until smooth. Stir in lemon juice, onion, salt and pepper. Cover and refrigerate for 30 minutes.

2. Gently stir sour cream into avocado mixture. Spoon into a serving bowl, surround with tortilla chips and serve.

NUTRITIONAL ANALYSIS	Energy	Protein	Carbohydrate	Fat	Iron
per tbsp (15 mL)	17 kcal	0.2 g	0.8 g	1.5 g	0.09 mg

**over 18
months**

Makes 32

Flavored Snacking Chips

*In this recipe, corn or flour tortillas (or pitas) become tasty crisp morsels
for between-meal bites. Make them in sizes that little fingers can handle.*

PREHEAT OVEN TO 425° F (220° C)
BAKING SHEET

4	corn or flour tortillas *or* pita bread halves	4
1/4 cup	vegetable oil	50 mL
1/2 tsp	garlic powder *or* onion powder	2 mL
1/2 tsp	herb blend	2 mL

1. Lightly brush corn or flour tortillas or pita halves with
    oil. Sprinkle with garlic powder and herbs. Cut each
    with scissors into 8 wedge-shaped pieces. Arrange in
    a single layer on baking sheet. Bake for 8 minutes or
    until crisp and golden brown. Allow to cool before
    storing in a tightly sealed container.

NUTRITIONAL ANALYSIS	Energy	Protein	Carbohydrate	Fat	Iron
per serving (4 chips)	93 kcal	1.4 g	8.5 g	5.9 g	0.40 mg

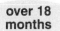

**over 18
months**

Makes 10 cups (2.5 L)

Snack Mix

1/4 cup	vegetable oil	50 mL
6 cups	chex-type cereal	1.5 L
8 oz	mini crackers (such as Ritz)	250 g
1	pkg (1 oz [28 g]) ranch-style salad dressing mix (powder)	1
2 to 3 tbsp	dried dill	25 to 45 mL

1. In a small bowl, heat oil in microwave for 45 to
    60 seconds until warm.

2. In a large bag, combine cereal, crackers, ranch
    powder and dill. Sprinkle with oil and shake.
    Store in an airtight container.

NUTRITIONAL ANALYSIS	Energy	Protein	Carbohydrate	Fat	Iron
per 1/4 cup (50 mL)	70 kcal	1.3 g	10.1 g	3.1 g	1.30 mg

over 18 months

Makes about 36 cookies

Old-Fashioned Chocolate Chip Cookies

PREHEAT OVEN TO 350° F (180° C)
COOKIE SHEET

1/ 3 cup	shortening	75 mL
1/3 cup	butter or margarine, softened	75 mL
1/2 cup	granulated sugar	125 mL
1/2 cup	brown sugar	125 mL
1	egg	1
1 tsp	vanilla extract	5 mL
1 1/2 cups	all-purpose flour	375 mL
1/2 tsp	salt	2 mL
1/2 tsp	baking soda	2 mL
3/4 cup	chocolate chips	175 mL

1. In a large bowl with an electric mixer, cream together shortening and butter. Add granulated sugar, brown sugar, egg and vanilla. Mix until smooth. Stir in flour, salt and baking soda. Fold in chocolate chips.

2. Drop dough in spoonfuls onto cookie sheet. Bake in preheated oven for 8 to 12 minutes or until browned.

NUTRITIONAL ANALYSIS	Energy	Protein	Carbohydrate	Fat	Iron
per cookie	95 kcal	0.9 g	11.8 g	5.2 g	0.44 mg

over 18
months

Makes about 30 cookies

Best Chocolate Chip and Oatmeal Cookies

PREHEAT OVEN TO 375° F (190° C)

BAKING SHEET, GREASED

1 cup	rolled oats	250 mL
1 cup	all-purpose flour	250 mL
1/4 tsp	salt	1 mL
1/2 tsp	baking powder	2 mL
1/2 tsp	baking soda	2 mL
1/2 cup	butter or margarine, softened	125 mL
1 cup	packed brown sugar	250 mL
1	egg	1
1/2 tsp	vanilla extract	2 mL
1 1/2 cups	semi-sweet chocolate chips	375 mL

1. In a large bowl, combine oats, flour, salt, baking powder and baking soda. Set aside.

2. In another large bowl with an electric mixer, combine butter, sugar, egg and vanilla; beat until smooth. Add flour mixture; mix well. Fold in chocolate chips. Spoon batter onto prepared cookie sheet, making 1-inch (2.5 cm) round balls. Bake in preheated oven for 8 to 10 minutes or until just browned.

NUTRITIONAL ANALYSIS	Energy	Protein	Carbohydrate	Fat	Iron
per cookie	133 kcal	1.5 g	17.8 g	6.9 g	0.82 mg

over 18 months

Makes about 48 cookies

Old-Fashioned Gingersnaps

Kitchen Tip

These cookies tend to burn quickly, so keep an eye on them while baking.

PREHEAT OVEN TO 350° F (180° C)

BAKING SHEET

3 cups	all-purpose flour	750 mL
2 tsp	baking soda	10 mL
1 tsp	ground ginger	5 mL
1 tsp	ground cinnamon	5 mL
1/2 tsp	salt	2 mL
1/2 tsp	ground cloves	2 mL
3/4 cup	margarine or shortening	175 mL
1 cup	packed brown sugar	250 mL
1	egg	1
3/4 cup	molasses	175 mL
1/2 cup	granulated sugar	125 mL

1. In a bowl, sift flour together with baking soda, ginger, cinnamon, salt and cloves.

2. In a large bowl with an electric mixer, beat margarine until creamy. Gradually add brown sugar. Beat in egg and molasses. Stir in flour mixture and mix well. Wrap dough in plastic wrap or waxed paper; refrigerate for about 1 hour or until firm enough to handle.

3. Shape dough into 1 1/2-inch (3.5 cm) balls and roll in the sugar. Place balls on cookie sheet 2 inches (5 cm) apart. Bake in preheated oven for 8 to 10 minutes or until browned. Cool on wire racks.

NUTRITIONAL ANALYSIS	Energy	Protein	Carbohydrate	Fat	Iron
per cookie	94 kcal	1.0 g	15.9 g	3.0 g	1.34 mg

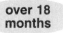
over 18 months

Makes about 48 cookies

Great Oatmeal Cookies

Kids love these cookies, as do adults.
Best of all, they're simple and quick to bake.

PREHEAT OVEN TO 350° F (180° C)
BAKING SHEET, GREASED

1 cup	butter or margarine, softened	250 mL
1/2 cup	granulated sugar	125 mL
3/4 cup	brown sugar	175 mL
1	egg	1
1/2 tsp	vanilla extract	2 mL
1/2 tsp	almond extract	2 mL
1 1/2 cups	all-purpose flour	375 mL
1/2 tsp	salt	2 mL
1 tsp	baking soda	5 mL
2 cups	rolled oatmeal	500 mL

1. In a bowl with an electric mixer, combine butter, granulated sugar, brown sugar, egg, vanilla and almond extract. Beat until smooth.

2. In another bowl, combine flour, salt, baking soda, and oatmeal. Add to butter mixture; mix well.

3. Spoon out about 1 tbsp (15 mL) dough and shape into a round ball. Place on baking sheet. Flatten with a moistened fork. Bake in preheated oven for about 12 minutes or until lightly browned.

NUTRITIONAL ANALYSIS	Energy	Protein	Carbohydrate	Fat	Iron
per cookie	86 kcal	1.1 g	10.6 g	4.5 g	0.81 mg

**over 18
months**

Serves 4 adults

Makes 20 baby servings

Apple Peach Crisp
and Oats

Kitchen Tip

If peaches are difficult to peel,
plunge into boiling water for
1 minute.

If you wish, replace peaches with
additional apples.

Delicious when served warm with vanilla ice cream.

PREHEAT OVEN TO 375° F (190° C)

8-INCH (2 L) CASSEROLE

7	medium apples, peeled and sliced	7
3	medium peaches, peeled and sliced	3
1/4 cup	granulated sugar	50 mL
1 tbsp	lemon juice	15 mL
2/3 cup	all-purpose flour	150 mL
2/3 cup	quick-cooking oats	150 mL
1/3 cup	packed brown sugar	75 mL
1/2 tsp	ground cinnamon	2 mL
1/4 cup	butter or margarine, melted	50 mL

1. Place apple and peach slices on bottom of casse-
    role. Sprinkle with sugar and lemon juice; toss to
    coat thoroughly.

2. In a bowl combine flour, oats, brown sugar and
    cinnamon. Pour melted butter over. Mix together
    to make a crumbly mixture. Sprinkle mixture
    evenly over fruit.

3. Bake in preheated oven for 45 minutes, or until
    fruit is softened and crumbly topping is crisp.

NUTRITIONAL ANALYSIS	Energy	Protein	Carbohydrate	Fat	Iron
per 1/4 cup (50 mL)	95 kcal	1.0 g	18.7 g	2.3 g	0.44 mg

Desserts

A B C D E F G H I J K L M N O P Q R S T U V W X Y Z

12 to 18 months

Makes 2 1/2 cups (625 mL)

Vanilla Cream

Variation

Raspberry Vanilla Parfait: Dissolve half a package of raspberry gelatin into 1/4 cup (50 mL) boiling water. Top it up to 1 cup (250 mL) with cold water. Cool. When the gelatin has almost set, layer the vanilla cream with the raspberry gelatin in parfait glasses. Refrigerate until set.

Serving Suggestion

Pour this cream over fresh fruit for dessert or serve plain on its own. You can also use whole milk in place of the evaporated milk.

3/4 cup	evaporated 2% milk	175 mL
1 3/4 cups	water	425 mL
1/4 cup	cornstarch	50 mL
1/4 cup	granulated sugar	50 mL
1/4 tsp	vanilla extract	1 mL

1. In a saucepan combine evaporated milk and water. Bring to a boil, stirring constantly. Remove from heat.

2. In a small bowl, combine cornstarch and sugar with 1 tbsp (15 mL) of the milk mixture. Stir back into milk in saucepan. Return to a boil and cook, stirring constantly, for 3 to 4 minutes or until thick. Add vanilla. Let cool before serving.

NUTRITIONAL ANALYSIS	Energy	Protein	Carbohydrate	Fat	Iron
per 1/4 cup (50 mL)	44 kcal	1.4 g	8.7 g	0.4 g	0.05 mg

Serves 6 adults

Makes 12 baby slices

Apple Pudding

PREHEAT OVEN TO 375° F (190° C)

9-INCH (23 CM) PIE PAN

4	medium baking apples, peeled, cored and sliced	4
1/3 cup	water	75 mL
1/4 cup	granulated sugar	50 mL
1/3 cup	butter *or* margarine	75 mL
1/3 cup	granulated sugar	75 mL
2	eggs	2
1 cup	all-purpose flour	250 mL
1 1/2 tsp	baking powder	7 mL
1/4 tsp	salt	1 mL
	Granulated sugar	

1. Place apples in pan with the water and the 1/4 cup (50 mL) granulated sugar. Bake in pre-heated oven for 10 minutes.

2. In a large bowl with an electric mixer, cream together butter and 1/3 cup (75 mL) sugar. Gradually beat in eggs. Stir in flour sifted with baking powder and salt. Spread mixture over hot apples; bake for another 35 to 40 minutes. Sprinkle with additional sugar before serving.

NUTRITIONAL ANALYSIS	Energy	Protein	Carbohydrate	Fat	Iron
per 1/4 cup (50 mL)	156 kcal	2.3 g	24.1 g	6.0 g	0.65 mg

Serves 4
Makes 1 cup (250 mL)

DESSERTS

Microwave Crème Brulée

Kitchen Tip

Use regular or 2% evaporated milk.

For even cooking, prepare in individual cups.

Serving Tip

For adults, sprinkle top of each dessert with 1 tsp (5 mL) brown sugar. Arrange cups on a baking pan; place under preheated broiler. Broil until sugar is melted and browned. Fresh fruit makes a nice garnish. (The crisp sugar topping is not suitable for children.)

This dessert is easily made in the microwave oven in one-quarter of the time required by conventional baking. It is readily handled by young eaters just learning to manage a spoon.

FOUR 1/3-CUP (75 ML) MICROWAVE-SAFE CUSTARD CUPS

1	can (6 oz [160 mL]) evaporated milk	1
1/3 cup	granulated sugar	75 mL
2	eggs	2
1 tsp	vanilla extract	5 mL

1. In a small microwavable bowl, combine milk and granulated sugar. Microwave at High for 1 minute or until hot. Stir to dissolve sugar.

2. In a second bowl, combine eggs and vanilla; beat until well mixed. Stir in hot milk mixture; pour into custard cups. Arrange cups in a circle in microwave oven; microwave at Medium for 2 minutes or until each cup shows signs of bubbling. (Do not overcook; desserts should still be slightly liquid, but will thicken on standing.) Allow to cool at room temperature. Chill until time to serve.

NUTRITIONAL ANALYSIS	Energy	Protein	Carbohydrate	Fat	Iron
per 1/4 cup (50 mL)	144 kcal	6.2 g	21.1 g	3.6 g	0.65 mg

12 to 18 months

Serves 6

Apple Bread Pudding

Kitchen Tip

Instead of apples, try other fruit in season, such as strawberries, raspberries, pears or peaches.

Apples, cinnamon and nutmeg elevate humble bread pudding to make this very special dessert. You can enhance it even more by adding a serving of Lemon or Vanilla Custard Sauce (see recipes, pages 264 and 265). Its soft texture is ideal for wee ones still lacking a full set of teeth.

PREHEAT OVEN TO 350° F (180° C)

6-CUP (1.5 L) SQUARE BAKING DISH

2 cups	2% milk	500 mL
1/3 cup	packed brown sugar	75 mL
1/2 tsp	ground cinnamon	2 mL
1/2 tsp	ground nutmeg	2 mL
2	eggs	2
1 tsp	vanilla extract	5 mL
2 cups	bread cubes	500 mL
2 tbsp	butter *or* margarine	25 mL
1	large apple, peeled, cored and thinly sliced (see Tip)	1

1. In bowl, whisk together milk, sugar, cinnamon, nutmeg, eggs and vanilla. Stir in bread and let stand for 10 minutes.

2. Meanwhile, place butter in baking dish and heat in oven until melted; swirl to cover bottom of dish. Pour in bread mixture. Top with apples, pushing slices down into bread mixture.

3. Bake in preheated oven for 40 minutes or until puffed and browned. Serve warm ensuring that infant portions have cooled to a safe temperature.

NUTRITIONAL ANALYSIS	Energy	Protein	Carbohydrate	Fat	Iron
per serving	177 kcal	5.8 g	22.5 g	7.2 g	1.06mg

12 to 18 months

Serves 4

Makes 2 1/4 cups (550 mL)

DESSERTS

Creamy Rice Pudding

Kitchen Tip

For all the creaminess that you expect from a great rice pudding, use Arborio rice for this recipe. But if you can't find any, conventional long grain rice will do the job. Just stay away from instant rice – it doesn't work very well.

Add vanilla to this or any other dessert after it has been removed from the heat. If added before, the vanilla flavor will evaporate.

Rice pudding has a long history of being one of the great "comfort" desserts. Traditionalists demand raisins in their rice pudding, but why not try cranberries for a change? Self-feeding little ones can easily cope with rice pudding. It sticks equally well to a spoon or to fingers.

3 cups	2% milk	750 mL
1/2 cup	Arborio or long grain rice (See Tip)	125 mL
1/4 cup	granulated sugar	50 mL
1	cinnamon stick	1
1/4 tsp	freshly gated nutmeg	1 mL
1/4 tsp	salt	1 mL
1 tsp	vanilla extract	5 mL
1/4 cup	chopped raisins *or* dried cranberries	50 mL

1. In a heavy saucepan over medium-high heat, combine milk, rice, sugar, cinnamon stick, nutmeg and salt. Bring to a boil. Reduce heat to low and cook, uncovered and stirring frequently, for 25 minutes or until rice is tender and creamy.

2. Remove and discard cinnamon stick. Stir in vanilla and raisins; cover and let stand for 10 minutes. Spoon into serving dishes and serve warm.

NUTRITIONAL ANALYSIS	Energy	Protein	Carbohydrate	Fat	Iron
per 1/4 cup (50 mL)	47 kcal	1.6 g	8.4 g	0.9 g	0.20 mg

12 to 18 months

Makes 3 1/2 cups (875 mL)

Mandarin Pudding

PREHEAT OVEN TO 350° F (180° C)

6-CUP (1.5 L) CASSEROLE, LIGHTLY GREASED

2 1/2 tbsp	butter *or* margarine	32 mL
2 1/2 tbsp	all-purpose flour	32 mL
1 1/4 cups	2% milk	300 mL
2	eggs, separated	2
1/4 cup	canned mandarin juice (see below)	50 mL
1/2 cup	granulated sugar	125 mL
1	can (10 oz [284 mL]) mandarin orange sections, drained, 1/4 cup (50 mL) juice reserved	1
2 tbsp	granulated sugar	25 mL

1. In a large saucepan over medium-high heat, melt butter. Add flour and cook, stirring, until bubbly. Remove from heat and gradually whisk in milk. Return to heat and bring to a boil, stirring constantly. Add egg yolks, reserved 1/4 cup (50 mL) mandarin juice, 1/2 cup (125 mL) sugar and mandarin sections (reserve some fruit for garnishing). Place mixture into casserole and bake in preheated oven for 15 to 20 minutes or until set.

2. In a separate bowl, beat egg whites until soft peaks form. Add 2 tbsp (25 mL) sugar and continue beating until stiff. Pipe meringue on top of pudding. Sprinkle with sugar and decorate with fruit.

3. Return pudding to oven and bake just until meringue is brown. Serve immediately.

NUTRITIONAL ANALYSIS	Energy	Protein	Carbohydrate	Fat	Iron
per 1/4 cup (50 mL)	91 kcal	1.9 g	13.7 g	3.3 g	0.29 mg

12 to 18 months

Makes 5 1/4 cups (1.375 L)

Baked Rice Pudding

This pudding is delicious served warm with whole or evaporated milk poured on top.

PREHEAT OVEN TO 375° F (190° C)

8-CUP (2 L) CASSEROLE

1/2 cup	chopped raisins	125 mL
4 cups	water	1 L
1 cup	rice	250 mL
1/2 cup	granulated sugar	125 mL
2	eggs, beaten	2
2 cups	2 % milk	500 mL
1 tbsp	butter *or* margarine	15 mL
	Ground cinnamon	

1. In a small bowl, cover raisins with hot water and allow to soak.

2. In a saucepan boil 4 cups (1 L) water. Add rice and cook for about 15 minutes. Drain.

3. Drain raisins. Add rice to casserole, along with sugar, eggs and raisins; mix well. Pour milk over. Top with small pieces of butter. Bake uncovered in preheated oven for about 1 hour or until crust is golden. Sprinkle with cinnamon just before serving.

NUTRITIONAL ANALYSIS	Energy	Protein	Carbohydrate	Fat	Iron
per 1/4 cup (50 mL)	90 kcal	2.2 g	17.0 g	1.6 g	0.30 mg

12 to 18 months

Makes 2 cups (500 mL)

Vanilla Pudding

Variation

To make this a chocolate pudding, add 3 tbsp (45 mL) cocoa to dry ingredients.

2 cups	2% milk, divided	500 mL
3 tbsp	cornstarch	45 mL
1/3 cup	granulated sugar	75 mL
1/4 tsp	salt	1 mL
1/2 tsp	vanilla extract	2 mL

1. In a double boiler, heat 1 3/4 cups (425 mL) of the milk over medium heat.

2. In a saucepan blend cornstarch, sugar, salt and remaining 1/4 cup (50 mL) milk. Gradually stir in heated milk from the double boiler; cook over medium heat, stirring constantly, until the mixture boils. Continue cooking for 1 minute. Remove saucepan from heat and stir in vanilla. Allow to cool before serving.

NUTRITIONAL ANALYSIS	Energy	Protein	Carbohydrate	Fat	Iron
per 1/4 cup (50 mL)	74 kcal	2.2 g	13.7 g	1.2 g	0.04 mg

12 to 18 months

Makes 12 slices

Kitchen Tip

Frost with Creamy Icing (see recipe, page 257) and decorate as desired.

Baby's First Birthday Cake

Here's a simple cake that's ideal for baby's first birthday.

PREHEAT OVEN TO 375° F (190° C)

TWO 9-INCH (2 L) ROUND CAKE PANS, GREASED AND FLOURED

1 cup	butter *or* margarine	250 mL
2 cups	granulated sugar	500 mL
4	eggs	4
3 cups	cake-and-pastry flour	750 mL
2 tsp	baking powder	10 mL
1/2 tsp	salt	2 mL
1 cup	2% milk	250 mL
1 tsp	vanilla extract	5 mL

1. In large bowl, cream together butter, sugar and eggs.

2. In another large bowl, sift together flour, baking powder and salt.

3. In a small bowl, combine milk and vanilla. Alternately add flour and milk mixtures to egg mixture; mix just until blended. Pour batter into prepared cake pans. Bake in preheated oven for 25 to 35 minutes or until toothpick inserted in center comes out clean.

NUTRITIONAL ANALYSIS	Energy	Protein	Carbohydrate	Fat	Iron
per slice (iced)	540 kcal	5.3 g	81.8 g	22.0 g	1.64 mg

Makes 1 cup (250 mL)

Creamy Icing

Kitchen Tip

If icing is too thin, add more confectioner's sugar. If icing is too thick, add more milk.

2 cups	confectioner's (icing) sugar	500 mL
1/4 cup	butter or margarine, softened	50 mL
1 tsp	vanilla extract	5 mL
3 to 4 tbsp	2% milk	45 to 60 mL

1. In a bowl with an electric mixer, cream together sugar and butter. Add vanilla. Slowly add sufficient milk to achieve desired consistency.

Makes enough for 1 cake

White Icing

5 tbsp	all-purpose flour, sifted	75 mL
1 cup	2% milk	250 mL
1 cup	butter *or* margarine	250 mL
1 cup	granulated sugar	250 mL
1 tsp	vanilla extract	5 mL

1. In a saucepan combine flour and milk. Bring to a boil and cook, stirring constantly, until thickened. Let cool for 1 hour.

2. In a large bowl with an electric mixer, combine butter, sugar and vanilla; beat until smooth. Beat in flour mixture. Spread onto cooled cake.

12 to 18 months

Makes one 24-slice cake

Spice-Swirl Pudding Cake

PREHEAT OVEN TO 350° F (180° C)

10-INCH (25 CM) TUBE PAN, GREASED

1/4 cup	firmly packed brown sugar	50 mL
1 tsp	ground cinnamon	5 mL
1/4 tsp	ground nutmeg	1 mL
1	pkg (4 oz [113 g]) vanilla instant pudding mix	1
1	pkg (15 1/4 oz [515 g]) yellow or white cake mix	1
4	eggs	4
1 cup	water	250 mL
1/4 cup	vegetable oil	50 mL

1. In a bowl combine brown sugar, cinnamon and nutmeg. Set aside.

2. In a large bowl with an electric mixer, combine pudding mix, cake mix, eggs, water and oil; blend for 2 minutes at medium speed.

3. Pour one-third of batter into prepared tube pan. Sprinkle with half of sugar mixture. Repeat layers, finishing with a layer of batter. Bake in preheated oven for 55 to 60 minutes or until a toothpick inserted in center of cake comes out clean. Let cool for 15 minutes, remove from pan and continue to cool on rack. When cool, frost with WHITE ICING (see recipe, page 257).

NUTRITIONAL ANALYSIS	Energy	Protein	Carbohydrate	Fat	Iron
per slice (iced)	266 kcal	2.5 g	29.5 g	13.7 g	0.72 mg

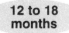

12 to 18 months

Makes 24 cupcakes

Carrot Cupcakes

Kitchen Tip

Enjoy these cupcakes on their own or with a cream cheese frosting of your choice.

PREHEAT OVEN TO 325° F (160° C)

12-CUP MUFFIN TIN, GREASED OR PAPER-LINED

2 cups	all-purpose flour	500 mL
2 cups	granulated sugar	500 mL
1 tsp	baking powder	5 mL
1 tsp	baking soda	5 mL
1 tsp	salt	5 mL
1 tsp	ground cinnamon	5 mL
3 cups	finely shredded carrots	750 mL
1 cup	vegetable oil	250 mL
4	eggs, slightly beaten	4

1. In a large bowl, combine flour, sugar, baking powder, baking soda, salt and cinnamon. Add shredded carrots, oil and eggs; beat until combined.

2. Pour batter into prepared cupcake tins and bake in preheated oven for 20 to 25 minutes or until toothpick inserted in center comes out clean. Cool before serving.

NUTRITIONAL ANALYSIS	Energy	Protein	Carbohydrate	Fat	Iron
per cupcake	212 kcal	2.3 g	27.4 g	10.7 g	0.73 mg

over 18 months

Makes 3 cups (750 mL)

DESSERTS

Spiced Semolina Pudding

PREHEAT OVEN TO 400° F (200° C)

4-CUP (1 L) CASSEROLE, GREASED

2 1/2 cups	2% milk	625 mL
3 tbsp	semolina	45 mL
1 tsp	ground allspice	5 mL
1/3 cup	granulated sugar	75 mL
	Grated zest of half lemon	
2	eggs, separated	2
1/4 cup	chopped currants	50 mL

1. In a saucepan over medium-high heat, combine milk, semolina and allspice. Bring to a boil and cook, stirring, until mixture thickens. Continue to cook for approximately 5 minutes. Remove saucepan from heat. Stir in sugar, zest, egg yolks and currants.

2. In a medium bowl, whisk egg whites until they are stiff; gently fold into pudding mixture.

3. Transfer mixture to prepared casserole and bake in preheated oven for about 20 minutes or until lightly brown.

NUTRITIONAL ANALYSIS	Energy	Protein	Carbohydrate	Fat	Iron
per 1/4 cup (50 mL)	69 kcal	3.1 g	10.0 g	2.0 g	0.34 mg

over 18 months

Makes one 24-slice cake

Banana Cake

This moist, delicious cake is a great way to use up overripe bananas.

Kitchen Tip

For a different flavor twist, try adding 1 cup (250 mL) chocolate chips.

PREHEAT OVEN TO 325° F (170° C)
9- BY 5-INCH (2 L) LOAF PAN

1 cup	butter or margarine, softened	250 mL
1 3/4 cups	granulated sugar	425 mL
4	eggs, beaten	4
2 tsp	vanilla extract	10 mL
3 cups	all-purpose flour	750 mL
2 tsp	baking powder	10 mL
2 tsp	baking soda	10 mL
1/2 tsp	salt	2 mL
1/2 tsp	ground allspice	2 mL
1/2 tsp	ground cinnamon	2 mL
5	ripe bananas	5

1. In a large bowl with an electric mixer, cream together butter and sugar. Beat in eggs and vanilla.

2. In another bowl, combine flour, baking powder, baking soda, salt, allspice and cinnamon. Stir into egg mixture. Add bananas and mix thoroughly. Transfer mixture to loaf pan.

3. Bake in preheated oven for 30 minutes. Increase temperature to 350° F (180° C) and bake for another 30 minutes.

NUTRITIONAL ANALYSIS	Energy	Protein	Carbohydrate	Fat	Iron
per slice	225 kcal	3.0 g	33.2 g	9.3 g	0.93 mg

over 18 months

Serves 6

Lemon Custard Pudding Cake

Kitchen Tip

Instead of a single baking dish, use 6 individual baking dishes and reduce baking time to 30 minutes.

Children really love the lemon flavor of this old-fashioned dessert. It never seems to go out of fashion.

PREHEAT OVEN TO 350° F (180° C)

8-CUP (2 L) BAKING DISH, LIGHTLY GREASED

1/3 cup	all-purpose flour	75 mL
1/3 cup	butter or margarine, melted	75 mL
1 1/2 cups	granulated sugar, divided	375 mL
4	eggs, separated	4
1 1/2 cups	2% milk	375 mL
	Grated zest of 1 lemon	
2 tbsp	lemon juice	25 mL

1. In a large bowl, combine flour, butter and 1 cup (250 mL) of the sugar. In a small bowl, beat egg yolks; add to flour mixture along with milk and zest. Mix well. Stir in lemon juice.

2. In another bowl, beat egg whites until stiff, but not dry. Gradually beat in remaining sugar until stiff peaks form. Fold into batter.

3. Pour batter into prepared baking dish. Place in a shallow pan of hot water and bake in preheated oven for 55 minutes or until lightly browned. Serve warm.

NUTRITIONAL ANALYSIS	Energy	Protein	Carbohydrate	Fat	Iron
per serving	400 kcal	7.1 g	61.9 g	14.8 g	1.13 mg

over 18 months

Serves 6

Makes 3 cups (750 mL)

Kitchen Tip

Use your favorite dried fruits such as apricots, pears, banana chips, prunes, dates or figs.

Fall Fruit Compote

The whole family will enjoy this flavorful compote of fall fruits and citrus. Inexpensive and easy to make, it keeps well in the refrigerator and can be frozen for longer storage.

2	large apples or pears, peeled, cored and sliced	2
1	medium orange	1
1	lemon	1
4 oz	dried mixed fruit (see Tip)	125 g
1/4 cup	granulated sugar	50 mL
3/4 cup	water	175 mL
1	cinnamon stick	1

1. Place apple slices in a saucepan. Remove large strips of zest from orange and lemon; add to apples. Peel orange, cut into chunks and add to apples. Squeeze lemon and measure 1 tbsp (15 mL) juice; add to apples along with dried fruit, sugar, water and cinnamon stick.

2. Bring mixture to a boil. Reduce heat to medium-low, cover and cook for 10 minutes or until fruit is tender. Remove orange and lemon strips, as well as cinnamon stick; discard. Allow to cool slightly. Serve at room temperature or cover and refrigerate for 4 hours or longer.

NUTRITIONAL ANALYSIS	Energy	Protein	Carbohydrate	Fat	Iron
per 1/4 cup (50 mL)	51 kcal	0.5 g	14.3 g	0.2 g	0.53 mg

over 18 months

Serves 3
Each makes 1 1/4 cups
(300 mL)

Kitchen Tip

Unused egg whites can be stored in the refrigerator for several days or frozen for several months.

Saucy Finishes

Make a dessert into something extra special with one of these sauces. Try them on Apple Bread Pudding (see recipe, page 251). They are also great on pancakes or over fresh fruit.

Vanilla Sauce

1/4 cup	granulated sugar	50 mL
1 tbsp	all-purpose flour	15 mL
Pinch	salt	Pinch
1 cup	2% milk, divided	250 mL
1	egg yolk (see Tip)	1
1 tbsp	butter *or* margarine	15 mL
1/2 tsp	vanilla extract	2 mL

1. In a small saucepan, combine sugar, flour and salt. Add 1/2 cup (125 mL) of the milk; stir until mixture is smooth. Whisk in remaining milk. Bring to a boil. Reduce heat and simmer, stirring constantly, for 2 minutes.

2. In a small bowl, stir egg yolk with a fork. Stir in some of the hot milk mixture and return to saucepan; cook, stirring constantly, for 1 minute (be careful to not boil). Remove from heat. Stir in butter and vanilla. Serve immediately.

NUTRITIONAL ANALYSIS	Energy	Protein	Carbohydrate	Fat	Iron
per 1 tbsp (15 mL)	25 kcal	0.6 g	3.0 g	1.1 g	0.07 mg

over 18 months

Makes 1 1/4 cups (300 mL)

Lemon Sauce

1/3 cup	granulated sugar	75 mL
2 tbsp	cornstarch	25 mL
1 tsp	grated lemon zest	5 mL
Pinch	salt	Pinch
1 cup	boiling water	250 mL
2 tbsp	butter *or* margarine	25 mL
2 tbsp	lemon juice	25 mL

1. In a small saucepan, combine sugar, cornstarch, lemon zest and salt. Gradually stir in boiling water. Cook over medium heat, stirring constantly, until sauce is clear and thickened. Remove from heat. Stir in butter and lemon juice. Serve immediately.

NUTRITIONAL ANALYSIS	Energy	Protein	Carbohydrate	Fat	Iron
per 1 tbsp (15 mL)	24 kcal	0.0 g	3.8 g	1.0 g	0.01 mg

over 18 months

Serves 8

Strawberry Angel Puff

Children will get a kick out of the name of this pleasant alternative to strawberry shortcake.

PREHEAT OVEN TO 425° F (230° C)

8 INDIVIDUAL OVENPROOF DISHES

Kitchen Tip

This dessert can be prepared to the end of Step 2, then frozen until ready to bake.

	Sauce	
2 cups	sliced strawberries	500 mL
2 tbsp	granulated sugar	25 mL
2 tbsp	frozen orange juice concentrate, thawed	25 mL
	Puff	
3	egg whites, at room temperature	3
1/8 tsp	cream of tartar	0.5 mL
3 tbsp	granulated sugar	45 mL
3 cups	torn bite-size pieces angel food cake (about half a 10 oz [300 g] cake)	750 mL
8	whole strawberries	8

1. Sauce: In a food processor, combine strawberries, sugar and orange juice; purée until smooth. Divide sauce between ovenproof bowls.

2. Puff: In a bowl with an electric mixer, beat egg whites and cream of tartar until foamy. Gradually beat in sugar until stiff peaks form. Fold in angel cake pieces. Divide mixture between dishes, mounding over sauce. Cover loosely with plastic wrap; freeze for several hours or until ready to bake.

3. Bake in preheated oven for 6 minutes or until meringue is golden brown. Allow to stand for several minutes before serving. Add a fresh whole strawberry as a garnish.

NUTRITIONAL ANALYSIS	Energy	Protein	Carbohydrate	Fat	Iron
per serving	120 kcal	3.9 g	22.0 g	2.1 g	0.65 mg

over 18 months

Serves 6 to 8

Fruit Clafouti Dessert

Kitchen Tip

For adults-only occasions, replace extract with rum or brandy.

Clafouti is a specialty of the Limousin region in central France. It features a thick egg batter which is poured over fresh fruit before baking. The result is sure to be a family favorite – and it is one of the easiest desserts you will ever make!

PREHEAT OVEN TO 350° F (180° C)

SHALLOW 8-CUP (2 L) BAKING DISH, GREASED

2 tbsp	butter *or* margarine	25 mL
6 cups	sliced fruit (such as peeled peaches, pears or apples	1.5 L
1/2 cup	2% milk	125 mL
1/3 cup	all-purpose flour	75 mL
1/3 cup	granulated sugar	75 mL
3	eggs	3
1 tsp	rum or brandy extract (see Tip)	5 mL
1/4 tsp	baking powder	1 mL
1 tbsp	granulated sugar	15 mL
1/2 tsp	ground cinnamon	2 mL

1. In a large microwavable container, melt butter on High for 20 seconds. Stir in fruit; microwave for 4 minutes or until fruit is barely tender. Transfer to prepared baking dish.

2. In a food processor or blender, combine milk, flour, 1/3 cup (75 mL) sugar, eggs, extract and baking powder; process until smooth. Pour over fruit mixture in baking dish, lifting slices with a fork to allow batter to run through. Sprinkle 1 tbsp (15 mL) sugar and cinnamon over top. Bake in preheated oven for 45 minutes or until knife inserted in center comes out clean. Serve warm.

NUTRITIONAL ANALYSIS	Energy	Protein	Carbohydrate	Fat	Iron
per serving	193 kcal	4.4 g	33.6 g	5.2 g	1.01 mg

over 18 months

Makes 4 cups (1 L)

Frozen Lemon Puff Dessert

Kitchen Tip

Spoon mixture into small popsicle molds and freeze for single servings.

It's amazing how many children seem to enjoy sucking on a fresh lemon. Here's the perfect dessert for them.

1/4 cup	granulated sugar	50 mL
2	eggs, separated	2
1/4 cup	lemon juice	50 mL
	Grated zest of 1 lemon	
1/2 cup	2% milk	125 mL
1 tsp	unflavored gelatin	5 mL
2 tbsp	granulated sugar	25 mL

1. In a small saucepan, combine 1/4 cup (50 mL) sugar, egg yolks, lemon juice, lemon zest and milk. Sprinkle gelatin over surface and let stand for 1 minute to soften.

2. Place saucepan over low heat and cook, stirring constantly, for about 5 minutes or until mixture is slightly thickened. Remove from heat and allow to cool slightly. Transfer to a metal bowl; cover and place in the freezer for 30 minutes or until mixture becomes thick; stir occasionally.

3. Beat egg whites with 2 tbsp (25 mL) sugar until stiff peaks form. Fold into chilled mixture, cover and return to freezer for several hours or until frozen.

NUTRITIONAL ANALYSIS	Energy	Protein	Carbohydrate	Fat	Iron
per 1/4 cup (50 mL)	31 kcal	1.2 g	4.7 g	0.9 g	0.16 mg

over 18 months

Makes 12 hats

Top Hats

These treats make a great dessert for a child's birthday party.

Kitchen Tip

Be sure to work quickly with this dessert so that chocolate melts without cooking.

12 PAPER CUPCAKE LINERS

3 oz	semi-sweet chocolate	75 mL
12	large marshmallows	12
12	Smarties or M&Ms *or* other candy	12

1. In a double boiler, heat chocolate until melted.

2. In cupcake liner, place about 1 tsp (5 mL) melted chocolate. Top with a marshmallow. Place a drop of melted chocolate on marshmallow and top with a Smartie. Refrigerate until the chocolate hardens.

NUTRITIONAL ANALYSIS	Energy	Protein	Carbohydrate	Fat	Iron
per top hat	66 kcal	0.5 g	10.8 g	2.9 g	0.32 mg

over 18 months

Makes 18 cup cakes

Banana Sour Cream Cup Cakes

Kitchen Tip

Since one of your muffin tins will be only half filled, fill empty cups with water to prevent the muffin tin from warping in the oven.

Banana and sour cream combine to give these cupcakes delicious flavor and moisture that lasts for several days, and will please the youngest appetite. One child we know loves to eat two cupcakes at a time, one held in each fist. If you're lucky, you may be offered a taste!

PREHEAT OVEN TO 350° F (180° C)

TWO 12-CUP MUFFIN TINS, NONSTICK OR PAPER-LINED

2 cups	cake-and-pastry flour	500 mL
2 tsp	baking powder	10 mL
1 tsp	baking soda	5 mL
1/4 cup	butter *or* margarine	50 mL
2/3 cup	granulated sugar	150 mL
2	eggs	2
1 cup	mashed bananas (about 2 small)	250 mL
2/3 cup	sour cream	150 mL
1/2 tsp	vanilla extract	2 mL

1. In a small bowl, combine flour, baking powder and soda. Set aside

2. In a large bowl with an electric mixer, cream butter until light and fluffy. Gradually beat in sugar, eggs and banana; blend until batter is smooth. Add flour mixture a bit at a time, alternating with sour cream and vanilla, stirring after each addition.

3. Spoon batter into muffin tins, leaving 6 cups empty (see Tip). Bake in preheated oven for 16 minutes or until firm to the touch

NUTRITIONAL ANALYSIS	Energy	Protein	Carbohydrate	Fat	Iron
per cupcake	129 kcal	2.1 g	21.3 g	4.1 g	0.70 mg

References

American Academy of Pediatrics. *Pediatric Nutrition Handbook, 4th ed.* Illinois: 1998.

American Academy of Pediatrics. *Caring For Your Baby & Young Child.* New York: Bantam Books, 1991.

American Academy of Pediatrics – Committee on Nutrition. *Hypoallergenic Infant Formulas.* New York: Bantam Books, 1991.

Arnon, S. S.; Midura T. F.; and Damus, K, et al. "Honey and other environmental risk factors for infant botulism." *Journal of Pediatrics* 1979; 94(2):331-336.

Baker, S. S.; Liptak, G. S.; Colletti, R. B.; et al. "Constipation in infants and children: evaluation and treatment." *Journal of Pediatric Gastroenterology and Nutrition* 1999; 29:612-626.

Bellioni-Businco, B.; Paganelli, R.; Lucotti, P.; Giampietro, P; Perborn, H; and Businco, L. "Allerginicity of goat's milk in children with cow's milk allergy." *Journal of Allergy and Clinical Immunology* 1999; 103:1191.

Belton, N. "Iron deficiency in infants and young children." *Prof Care Mother Child* 1995; 5:69-71.

Bhan, M. K.; Arora, N. K.; Khoshoo, V.; et al. "Comparison of a lactose-free cereal-based formula and cow's milk in infants and children with acute gastroenteritis." *Journal of Pediatric Gastroenterology and Nutrition* 1988; 7(2):208-213.

Canadian Pediatric Society. "Breastfeeding and Vitamin D." Fact sheet. February, 1999.

Canadian Pediatric Society. "Criteria for labeling infant formulas as 'hypoallergenic.'" *Canadian Medical Association Journal.* 1994; 150(6):883-884.

City of Toronto Department of Public Health. "Baby teeth are important." Fact sheet.

City of Toronto Department of Public Health "Growing up: how your dental needs change." Fact sheet.

City of Toronto Department of Public Health "How to prevent choking in children." Fact sheet.

Cook, D. A. "Nutrient levels in infant formulas: technical considerations." *Journal of Nutrition* 1989;119(12 Suppl):1773-1777.

Deeming, S. B. and Weber, C.W. "Trace minerals in commercially prepared baby foods." *Journal of the American Dietetic Association* 1979; 75:149-151.

Deheeger, M.; Rolland-Cacherea, M. F.; Pequignot, F.; et al. "Changes in food intake in 2-year-old children between 1973 and 1986." *Annals of Nutrition and Metabolism* 1991; 35:132-140.

Dennison, B. A. "Fruit juice consumption by infants and children: a review." *Journal of the American College of Nutrition* 1996; 15:4S-11S.

Dennison, B. A.; Rockwell, H. L.; and Baker, S. L. "Excess fruit juice consumption by preschool-aged children is associated with short stature and obesity." *Pediatrics* 1997; 99(1):15-22.

Dennison, B.A.; Rockwell, H. L.; and Baker, S. L. "Fruit and vegetable intake in young children." *Journal of the American College of Nutrition* 1998; 17:371-378.

Doucette, R. and Dwyer, J. T. "Is fruit juice a 'no-no' in children's diets?" *Nutrition Reviews* 2000; 58:180-183.

Dusdieker, L. B.; Getchel, J. P.; and Liarakos, T. M. "Nitrate in baby foods." *Archives of Pediatrics and Adolescent Medicine* 1994; 148:490-494.

Ellison, R. C.; Singer, M. R.; Moore, L. L.; et al. "Current caffeine intake of young children: amount and sources." *Journal of the American Dietetic Association* 1995; 95:802-804.

Filer, L. J. "Modified food starch: an update." *Journal of the American Dietetic Association* 1988; 88(3):342-344.

Finberg, L. "Modified fat diets: do they apply to infancy?" *Journal of Pediatrics* 1990; 117(2):S132-133.

Fomon, S. J. and Ekstrand, J. "Fluoride intake by infants." *Journal of Public Health Dentistry* 1999; 59:229-234.

Fontana, M.; Bianchi, C.; and Cataldo, F. "Bowel frequency in healthy children." *Acta Pediatrica Scandinavia* 1989; 78:682-684.

Friel, J. K.; Andrews, W. L.; Edgesombe, C; et al. "Eighteen-month follow-up of infants fed evaporated milk formula." *Canadian Journal of Public Health* 1999; 90:240-243.

Gibson, S. A. "Iron intake and iron status of preschool children: associations with breakfast cereals, vitamin C and meat." *Public Health Nutrition* 1999;2:521-528.

Gibson, S. A. "Breakfast cereal consumption in young children: associations with non-milk extrinsic sugars and caries experience: further analysis of data from the UK national diet and nutrition survey of children aged 1.5-4.5 years." *Public Health Nutrition* 2000; 227-232.

Grand, R. J.; Watkins, J. B.; and Torti, F. M. "Progress in gastroenterology. Development of the human gastrointestinal tract: a review." *Gastroenterology* 1976; 70(5);790-810.

Grunwaldt, E.; Bates, T.; and Guthrie, D. "The onset of sleeping through the night in infancy." *Pediatrics* 1960; October:667-668.

Guthrie and Piccano: *Human Nutrition.*

Haaf, W. "Clearing the Airways: How to protect your child from choking." *Today's Parent* August 2000: 34-38.

Health Canada. *A Multicultural Perspective of Breastfeeding in Canada.* Minister of Public Works and Government Services, Ottawa, 1997.

Health Canada. *Family-Centered Maternity and Newborn Care: National Guidelines.* Minister of Public Works and Government Services, Ottawa, 2000.

Hediger, M. L.; Overpeck, M. D.; Ruan, W. J.; and Troendle, J. F. "Early infant feeding and growth status of US-born infants and children aged 4-71 mo: analyses from the third National Health and Nutrition Examination Survey, 1988-94." *American Journal of Clinical Nutrition* 2000;72(1):159-167.

Henriksen, C.; Eggesbo, M.; Halvorsen, R.; and Botten, G. "Nutrient intake among two-year – old children on cow's milk-restricted diets." *Acta Pediatrica Scandinavia* 2000; 89:272-278.

Holliday, M. A.; "Is blood pressure in later life affected by events in infancy?" *Pediatric Nephrology* 1995; 9:663-666.

Hyams, J. S.; Etienne, N. L.; Leichtner, A. M.; and Theuer, R. C. "Carbohydrate malabsorption following fruit juice ingestion in young children." *Pediatrics* 1988; 82:64-68.

Hyams, J. S.; Treem, W. R.; Etienne, N. L.; et al. "Effect of infant formulas on stool characteristics of young infants." *Pediatrics* 1995; 95:50-54

Iacono, G.; Cavataio, F; Montalto, G.; et al. "Intolerance of cow's milk and chronic constipation in children." *New England Journal of Medicine* 1998; 339:1100-1104

Illingworth, R. S. *The Normal Child*, 10th ed. New York: Churchill Livingstone, 1991.

Johnsen, D. and Nowjack-Raymer, R. "Baby bottle tooth decay (BBTD): issues, assessment , and an opportunity for the nutritionist." *Perspectives in Practice* 1989; 89:1112-1116

Johnsen, D. C.; Gerstenmaier, J. H.; Schwartz, E.; et al. "Background comparisons of pre-3 1/2-year-old children with nursing caries in four practice settings." *Pediatric Dentistry* 1984; 6:50-54.

Joint Working Group of the Canadian Paediatric Society and Health Canada. *Nutrition Recommendations Update…Dietary Fat and Children.* Ottawa, 1993.

Joint Working Group of the Canadian Paediatric Society, Dietitians of Canada and Health Canada. *Nutrition for Healthy Term Infants.* Ottawa, 1998.

Joint Working Group of the Canadian Paediatric Society, Dietitians of Canada and Health Canada. *Question and Answer Document as a follow-up to "Nutrition for Healthy Term Infants."* Ottawa, 1999.

Kerr, C. M.; Reisinger, K. S.; and Plankey, F. W. "Sodium concentration of homemade baby foods." *Pediatrics* 1978; 62(3):331-335.

Klish, W. J. *Dietary fats in children: the American perspective.* Heinz Institute of Nutritional Sciences (HINS) Articles.

Koivisto Hursti, U. K. "Factors influencing children's food choice. *Annals of Medicine* 1999; 31:26-32.

Lambert-Lagacé, L. *Feeding Your Baby in the Nineties.* Toronto: Stoddart Publishing, 1992.

Laquatra, I. M. *Herbal remedies: cause or cure of ailments?* HINS Articles.

Lebenthal, E. "Impact of digestion and absorption in the weaning period on infant feeding practices." *Pediatrics* 1985; 75(suppl):207-213.

Lebenthal, E. "Use of modified food starches in infant nutrition." *American Journal of Disease in Children* 1978; 132:850-852.

Lebenthal, E.; Lee, P. C.; and Heitlinger, L. A. "Impact of development of the gastrointestinal tract on infant feeding." *Journal of Pediatrics* 1983; 102(1):1-9.

Lebenthal, E. and Shwachman, H. "The pancreas - Development, adaptation and malfunction in infancy and childhood. *Clinical Gastroenterology* 1977; 6(2):397-413.

Legius, E.; Proesmans, W.; Eggermont, E.; et al. "Rickets due to dietary calcium deficiency." *European Journal of Pediatrics* 1989; 148:784-785.

Lifschitz, C. H. and Abrams, S. A. "Addition of rice cereal to formula does not impair mineral bioavailability." *Journal of Pediatric Gastroenterology and Nutrition* 1998; 26:175-178.

Lozoff, B.; Jimenez, E.; Hagen, J.; et al. "Poorer behavioural and developmental outcome more than 10 years after treatment for iron deficiency in infancy." *Pediatrics* 2000; 105:E51.

Macknin, M. L.; VanderBrug Medendorp, S.; Maier, M. C. "Infant sleep and bedtime cereal." *American Journal of Disease in Children* 1989; 143:1066-1068.

Martinez , C.; Fox, T.; Eagles, J; and Fairweather-Tait, S. "Evaluation of iron bioavailability in infant weaning foods fortified with heme concentrate." *Journal of Pediatric Gastroenterology and Nutrition* 1998; 27:419-424.

Martinez, G. A. and Ryan, A. S. "Nutrient intake in the Untied States during the first 12 months of life." *Journal of American Dietetic Association* 1985; 85:826-830.

McVeagh, P. "Eating and nutritional problems in children." *Australian Family Physician* 2000; 29:735-740.

Mehta, K. C.; Specker, B. L.; Bartholmey, S.; et al. "Trial on timing of introduction to solids and food type on infant growth." *Pediatrics* 1998; 102(3):569-573.

Melina, V.; Davis, B.; and Harrison, V. *Becoming Vegetarian.* Toronto: Macmillan Canada, 1994.

Mennella, J. A. and Beauchamp, G. K. "Maternal diet alters the sensory qualities of human milk and the nursling's behavior." *Pediatrics* 1991; 88(4):737-743.

Mohrbacher, N. and Stock, J. *The Breastfeeding Answer Book*, revised edition. La Leche League International, 1997.

Neander, W. L. and Morse, J. M. "Tradition and change in the northern Alberta woodlands Cree: implications for infant feeding practice." *Canadian Journal of Public Health* 1989; 80:190-194.

Niinikoski, H.; Lapinleimu, H.; Viikari, J; et al. "Growth until 3 years of age in a prospective, randomized trial of a diet with reduced saturated fat and cholesterol." *Pediatrics* 1997; 99(5):687-694.

Nutrition Committee, Canadian Paediatric Society. "Megavitamin and megamineral therapy in childhood." *Canadian Medical Association Journal* 1990;143:1009-1013

Nutrition Committee, Canadian Paediatric Society. "Meeting the iron needs of infants and young children: an update." *Canadian Medical Association Journal* 1991; 144:1451-1454.

Nutrition Committee, Canadian Paediatric Society. "Oral rehydration therapy and early refeeding in the management of childhood gastroenteritis." *Canadian Journal of Paediatrics* 1994;1:160-164.

Nutrition Committee, Canadian Paediatric Society. "The use of fluoride in infants and children." *Paediatrics Child Health* 1996;1:131-134.

Oken, E. and Lightdale, J. R. "Updates in pediatric nutrition." *Current Opinion Pediatrics* 2000;12:282-290.

Picciano, M. F.; Smiciklas-Wright, H.; Birch, L. L.; et al. "Nutritional guidance is needed during dietary transition in early childhood." *Pediatrics* 2000; 106:109-114.

Pollock, I. and Warner, J. O. "Effect of artificial food colours on childhood behaviour." *Archives of Disease in Childhood* 1990; 65:74-77.

Riordan, J. and Auerbach, K. *Breastfeeding and Human Lactation,* 2nd ed. Jones and Bartlett Publishers, 1999.

Roberts, S. B. and Heyman, M. B. "Micronutrient shortfalls in young children's diets: common, and owing to inadequate intakes both at home and at child care centers." *Nutrition Reviews* 2000; 58:27-29.

Saarinen, K. M. and Savilahti, E. "Infant feeding patterns affect the subsequent immunological features in cow's milk allergy." *Clinical and Experimental Allergy* 2000; 30:400-406.

Shatenstein, B. and Ghadirian, P. "Influences on diet, health behaviours and their outcome in select ethnocultural and religious groups." *Nutrition* 1998; 14:223-30.

Short, R. V. "What the breast does for the baby, and what the baby does for the breast." *Australia and New Zealand Journal of Obstetrics and Gynaecology* 1994; 34:262-264.

Singhal, A.; Morely, R.; Abbott, R.; et al. "Clinical safety of iron fortified formulas." *Pediatrics* 1999; 103:58-64.

Skinner, J. D.; Carruth, B. R.; Moran, J. III; et al. "Fruit juice is not related to children's growth." *Pediatrics* 2000; 105(3):e38-44.

Smith, M. M. and Lifshitz, F. "Excess fruit juice consumption as a contributing factor in nonorganic failure to thrive." *Pediatrics* 1994; 93:438-443.

Stuphen, J. L. and Dillard, V. L. "Medium chain triglyceride in the therapy of gastroesophageal reflux." *Journal of Pediatric Gastroenterology and Nutrition* 1992; 14(1):38-40.

Tunnessen, W. W. and Oski, F. A. "Consequences of starting whole cow milk at 6 months of age." *Journal of Pediatrics* 1987; 111:813-816.

Van Den Boom, S.; Kimber, A. C.; and Morgan, J. B. "Nutritional composition of home-prepared baby foods in Madrid. Comparison with commercial products in Spain and home-made meals in England." *Acta Paediatrica* 1997; 86(1):57-62.

Vickerstaff-Joneja, J. *Managing Food Allergy & Intolerance: A Practical Guide.* 1995

Willows, N. D.; Morel, J.; and Gray-Donald, K. "Prevalence of anemia among James Bay Cree infants of northern Quebec." *Canadian Medical Association Journal* 2000; 162:323-326.

Wilson, N. and Scott, A. "A double-blind assessment of additive intolerance in children using a 12 day challenge period at home." *Clinical and Experimental Allergy* 1989; 19:267-272.

Wolraich, M. L.; Lindgren, S. D.; Stumbo, P. J.; et al. "Effects of diets high in sucrose or aspartame on the behavior and cognitive performance of children." *New England Journal of Medicine* 1994; 330:301-307.

Worthington-Roberts, B. S. and Rodwell Williams, S. *Nutrition Throughout the Life Cycle*, 3rd ed. St. Louis: Mosby Year Book Inc., 1996.

Yeung, D. L. "Nutritional adequacy of commercial baby foods." *J Assoc Off Anal Chem* 1982; 65(6):1500-1504.

Yeung, D. L.; Hall, J.; Leung, M.; and Pennell, M. D. "Sodium intakes of infants from 1 to 18 months of age." *Journal of American Dietetic Association* 1982; 80(3):242-242.

Yeung, D. L.; Pennell, M.D.; Leung, M.; and Hall, J. "Commercial or homemade baby food?" *Canadian Medical Association Journal* 1982; 126:113.

Yeung, G. S. and Zlotkin, S. H. "Efficacy of meat and iron-fortified commercial cereal to prevent iron depletion in cow milk-fed infants 6 to 12 months of age: a randomized controlled trial." *Canadian Journal of Public Health* 2000; 91:263-267.

Young, B. and Drewett, R. "Eating behaviour and its variability in 1-year-old children." *Appetite* 2000; 35:171-177.

Ziegler, E. E. and Fomon, S. J. "Lactose enhances mineral absorption in infancy." *Journal of Pediatric Gastroenterology and Nutrition* 1983;2:288-294

Zwiauer, K. F. "Prevention and treatment of overweight and obesity in children and adolescents." *European Journal of Pediatrics* 2000;159(Suppl1):S56-S68

RECOMMENDED WEB SITES

www.dietitians.ca A professional association for Registered Dietitians in Canada

www.canadian-health-network.ca Provides Internet access for credible health information.

www.sickkids.on.ca The Hospital for Sick Children, Toronto's pediatric hospital.

www.cda-adc.ca Canadian Dental Association, a professional association for Canadian dentists.

www.aap.org American Academy of Pediatrics, a professional association for American pediatricians.

www.cps.ca Canadian Pediatric Society, a professional association for Canadian pediatricians.

www.eatright.org American Dietetic Association, a professional association of dietitians in the U.S.A.

www.motherrisk.org Motherrisk, provides information on drug interactions and breastfeeding infants, etc.

www.specialtyfoodshop.com Specialty Food Shop, located at the Hospital for Sick Children in Toronto, providing food products for special diets, along with nutritional information.

www.heinzbaby.com Heinz Baby Foods, a Canadian site with 1-800-USA-BABY number for U.S. consumers

www.gerber.com Gerber Baby Foods.

www.beechnut.com Beech Nut Foods.

Sites specializing in providing information on infant formulas:

www.wyethnutritionals.com Wyeth

www.ross.com/html/unifiedsite.cfm Ross

www.meadjohnson.com Mead Johnson

www.verybestbaby.com Nestle

Index